WOMEN
AND
HEALTH

TODAY'S EVIDENCE
TOMORROW'S AGENDA

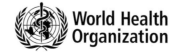 World Health
Organization

WHO Library Cataloguing-in-Publication Data:

Women and health : today's evidence tomorrow's agenda.

1.Women's health. 2.Women's health services - trends. 3.Life change events. 4.Health status indicators.
5.Social justice. 6.Gender identity. 7.Public policy. 8.World health. 9.Developing countries.
I.World Health Organization.

ISBN 978 92 4 156385 7   (NLM classification: WA 309)

Acknowledgements

This report was produced under the overall direction of Assistant Directors-General Tim Evans and Daisy Mafubelu. The editorial team members were, in alphabetical order, Carla AbouZahr, Isabelle de Zoysa and Claudia García Moreno. Valuable inputs were provided by Ties Boerma, Andrew Cassels, Susan Holck, Colin Mathers and Thomson Prentice.

Contributions were received from: Jonathan Abrahams, Fiona Adshead, Adelio Antunes, Timothy Armstrong, Gini Arnold, Parijat Baijal, Anand Balachandran, John Beard, Douglas Bettcher, Michel Beusenberg, Paul Bloem, Monika Blössner, Sophie Bonjour, Cynthia Boschi-Pinto, Francesco Branca, Nathalie Broutet, Marie-Noel Brune, Tony Burton, Alexander Butchart, Txema Calleja, Diarmid Campbell-Lundrum, Guy Carrin, Andrew Cassels, Somnath Chatterji, Rudi Coninx, Melanie Cowan, Catherine d'Arcanques, Mercedes de Onis, Bruce Dick, Tarun Dua, Varatharajan Durairaj, David Evans, Jane Ferguson, Daniela Fuhr, Lisa Garbus, Peter Ghys, Philip Glaziou, Fiona Gore, Rifat Hossein, Ahmadreza Hosseinpoor, Mie Inoue, Véronique Joseph, Mary Kay Kindhauser, Evelyn Kortum, Tanya Kuchenmuller, Jennifer Lee, Sun Goo Lee, Wim Van Lerberghe, Doris Ma Fat, José Martines, Elizabeth Mason, Pamela Sabina Mbabazi, Christopher Mikton, Charles Mock, Nirmala Naidoo, Francis Ndowa, Joerdis Ott, Heather Papowitz, Razia Pendse, Judy Polsky, Yongyuth Pongsupap, Vladimir Poznyak, Annette Prüss-Üstün, Eva Rehfuess, Chen Reis, Leanne Riley, Lisa Rogers, Ritu Sadana, Shekhar Saxena, Lale Say, George Schmid, Archana Narendra Shah, Iqbal Shah, Ferid Shannoun, Kurup Anand Sivasankara, Amani Siyam, Yves Souteyrand, Marcus Stalhofer, Claudia Stein, Gretchen Stevens, Joanna Tempowski, Shyam Thapa, Andreas Ullrich, Constanza Vallenas, Annette Verster, Susan Wilburn, Sachiyo Yoshida and Dongbao Yu.

Valuable comments were provided by Mahmoud Fatallah, Sharon Fonn, Adrienne Germain, Piroska Ostlin, Sundari Ravindran, Sheila Tlou and Tomris Türmen.

Special thanks go to the Department of Health Care Policy, Harvard Medical School – Robert Jin, Ronald C. Kessler and Nancy Sampson – for the analysis of women and mental ill-health data.

Further writing support was provided by Gary Humphries and Diane Summers. The report was edited by David Bramley and proof-read by Diana Hopkins. The index was prepared by June Morrison. Design and graphics were by Steve Ewart and Christophe Grangier. Print and web versions were prepared by Gael Kernen. Production editing by Melanie Lauckner. Administrative support in preparation of the report was provided by Sue Piccolo.

WHO is grateful to the Aspen Institute's Realizing Rights: Ethical Globalization Initiative for financial support to the production and dissemination of this report.

Printed in Switzerland

WOMEN AND HEALTH

Foreword

When I took office in 2007, I asked that my performance be judged by results as measured by the health of women and of the people of Africa. My commitment to these populations is a reaffirmation of WHO's long history of reaching out to those in greatest need and to redressing health inequalities and their determinants.

The Millennium Development Goals and other global commitments have focused primarily on the entitlements and needs of women. The current financial crisis and economic downturn make this focus even more urgent; protecting and promoting the health of women is crucial to health and development – not only for the citizens of today but also for those of future generations.

This report reviews evidence on the health issues that particularly affect girls and women throughout their life course. Despite considerable progress over the past two decades, societies are still failing women at key moments in their lives. These failures are most acute in poor countries, and among the poorest women in all countries. Not everyone has benefited equally from recent progress and too many girls and women are still unable to reach their full potential because of persistent health, social and gender inequalities and health system inadequacies.

This report does not offer a comprehensive analysis of the state of women and health in the world. The data and evidence that are available are too patchy and incomplete for this to be possible. Indeed, one of the striking findings of the report is the paucity of statistics on key health issues that affect girls and women. But the report does bring together what is currently known and identifies areas where new data need to be generated, available data compiled and analysed, and research undertaken to fill critical gaps in the evidence base.

In presenting this report, it is my hope that it will serve to stimulate policy dialogue at country, regional and global levels, to inform actions by countries, agencies, and development partners, and to draw attention to innovative strategies that will lead to real improvements in the health and lives of girls and women around the world.

Dr Margaret Chan
Director-General
World Health Organization

Introduction

This report uses currently available data to take stock of the health of girls and women around the world and to draw attention to the consequences and costs of failing to address health issues at appropriate points in their lives.

The report is structured around a life course divided into stages that have particular relevance for health – early childhood (from birth to nine years), adolescence (from 10 to 19 years), adulthood (from 20 to 59 years, and including the reproductive ages of 15–44 years) and older age (from 60 years onwards).[a] While many of the factors that affect the health of the girl child, the female adolescent, the adult and the older woman do not fit neatly or exclusively into these stages, the approach fosters a deeper understanding of how interventions in childhood, through adolescence, during the reproductive years and beyond affect health later in life and across the generations.

The data in this report are largely drawn from WHO databases and publications, and from publications of other United Nations agencies. Readers should consult these sources for further information on data compilation and methods of analysis. Main sources are referenced in the text. While bringing together a wealth of evidence, the report does not set out to be comprehensive; indeed, it points to significant gaps in knowledge relating to women's health.

While in some cases the report compares women with men, for the most part it draws attention to the differences in health and health care that girls and women face in different settings. The report highlights the interplay of biological and social determinants of women's health and draws attention to the role of gender inequality in increasing exposure and vulnerability to risk, limiting access to health care and information, and influencing health outcomes.

The report notes the importance of women's multiple contributions to society in both their productive and reproductive roles, and both as consumers and – just as importantly – as providers of health care. In recognition of this, the report calls for primary health care reforms to be implemented in ways that ensure that health systems better meet the needs of girls and women.

---

a These age groupings have been identified on the basis of health issues and needs and do not necessarily correspond to United Nations definitions.

EXECUTIVE SUMMARY

Overview

This is a report on women and health – both women's health needs and their contribution to the health of societies. Women's health has long been a concern for WHO but today it has become an urgent priority. This report explains why. Using current data, it takes stock of what we know *now* about the health of women throughout their lives and across the different regions of the world.

Highlighting key issues – some of which are familiar, others that merit far greater attention – the report identifies opportunities for making more rapid progress. It points to areas in which better information – plus policy dialogue at national, regional and international levels – could lead to more effective approaches. The report shows the relevance of the primary health care reforms set out in *The world health report 2008: primary health care – now more than ever*, laying particular emphasis on the urgent need for more coherent political and institutional leadership, visibility and resources for women's health, to enable us to make progress in saving the lives and improving the health of girls and women in the coming years. Finally, it sets out what the implications are in terms of data collection, analysis and dissemination.

The life-course approach taken in this report fosters a deeper understanding of how interventions in childhood, through adolescence, during the reproductive years and beyond, affect health later in life and across the generations. It also highlights the interplay of biological and social determinants of women's health, and draws attention to the role of gender inequality in increasing exposure and vulnerability to risk, limiting access to health care and information, and impacting on health outcomes. While the report calls for greater attention to health problems that affect only women – such as cervical cancer and the health risks associated with pregnancy and childbirth – it also shows that women's health needs go beyond sexual and reproductive concerns.

The report draws attention to the consequences and costs of failing to address health issues at the appropriate points of women's lives. In a world with an ageing population, the challenge is to prevent and manage the risk factors of today to ensure that they do not lead to the chronic health problems of tomorrow.

The life-course approach reveals the importance of women's multiple contributions to society – in both their productive and reproductive roles, as consumers and, just as importantly, as providers of health care. It is in recognition of this fact that the report calls for reforms to ensure that women become key agents in health-care provision – centrally involved in the design, management and delivery of health services.

Key findings

1. Widespread and persistent inequities

Disparities between women and men

While women and men share many similar health challenges, the differences are such that the health of women deserves particular attention. Women generally live longer than men because of both biological and behavioural advantages. But in some settings, notably in parts of Asia, these advantages are overridden by gender-based discrimination so that female life expectancy at birth is lower than or equal to that of males.

Moreover, women's longer lives are not necessarily healthy lives. There are conditions that only women experience and whose potentially negative impact only they suffer. Some of these – such as pregnancy and childbirth – are not diseases, but biological and social processes that carry health risks and require health care. Some health challenges affect both women and men, but have a greater or different impact on women and so require responses that are tailored specifically to women's needs. Other conditions affect women and men more or less equally, but women face greater difficulties in getting the health care they need. Furthermore, gender-based inequalities – for example in education, income and employment – limit the ability of girls and women to protect their health.

Differences between high- and low-income countries

While there are many commonalities in the health challenges facing women around the world, there are also striking differences due to the varied conditions in which they live. At every age, women in high-income countries live longer and are less likely to suffer from ill-health and premature mortality than those in low-income countries. In richer countries, death rates for children and young women are very low, and most deaths occur after 60 years of age. In poorer countries, the picture is quite different: the population is on average younger, death rates among children are higher, and most female deaths occur among girls, adolescents and younger adult women. The most striking difference between rich and poor countries is in maternal mortality – 99% of the more than half a million maternal deaths every year happen in developing countries. Not surprisingly, the highest burden of morbidity and mortality – particularly in the reproductive years – is concentrated in the poorest and often the institutionally weakest countries, particularly those facing humanitarian crises.

Inequalities within countries

Within countries, the health of girls and women is critically affected by social and economic factors, such as access to education, household wealth and place of residence. In almost all countries, girls and women living in wealthier households have lower levels of mortality and higher use of health-care services than those living in the poorest households. Such differences are not confined to developing countries but are found in the developed world.

2. Sexuality and reproduction are central to women's health

Women's health during the reproductive or fertile years (between the ages of 15 and 49 years) is relevant not only to women themselves, but also has an impact on the health and development of the next generation. Many of the health challenges during this period are ones that only young girls and women face. For example, complications of pregnancy and childbirth are the leading cause of death in young women aged between 15 and 19 years old in developing countries. Globally, the leading cause of death among women of reproductive age is HIV/AIDS. Girls and women are particularly vulnerable to HIV infection due to a combination of biological factors and gender-based inequalities, particularly in cultures that limit women's knowledge about HIV and their ability to protect themselves and negotiate safer sex. The most important risk factors for death and disability in this age group in low- and middle-income countries are lack of contraception and unsafe sex. These result in unwanted pregnancies, unsafe abortions, complications of pregnancy and childbirth, and sexually transmitted infections including HIV. Violence is an additional significant risk to women's sexual and reproductive health and can also result in mental ill-health and other chronic health problems.

3. The toll of chronic diseases, injuries and mental ill-health

While the sexual and reproductive health needs of women are generally well known, they also face other important health challenges.

Road traffic injuries are among the five leading causes of death for adolescent girls and women of reproductive age in all WHO regions – except for South-East Asia, where burns are the third leading cause of death. While many are the result of cooking accidents, some are homicides or suicides, often associated with violence by an intimate partner. More research is needed to better understand the underlying causes of these deaths and to identify effective prevention strategies.

Suicide is among the leading causes of death for women between the ages of 20 and 59 years globally and the second leading cause of death in the low- and middle-income countries of the WHO Western Pacific Region. Suicidal behaviour is a significant public health problem for girls and women worldwide. Mental health problems, particularly depression, are major causes of disability for women of all ages. While the causes of mental ill-health may vary from one individual to another, women's low status in society, their burden of work and the violence they experience are all contributing factors.

For women over 60 years of age in low-, middle- and high-income countries, cardiovascular disease and stroke are major killers and causes of chronic health problems. Another significant cause of death and disability is chronic obstructive pulmonary disease, which has been linked to women's exposure to smoke and indoor air pollution largely as a result of their household roles. For many women, ageing is accompanied by loss of vision – every year, more than 2.5 million older women go blind. Much of this burden of disability could be avoided if they had access to the necessary care, particularly surgery for cataracts. In low-income countries, trachoma is a significant, but preventable, cause of blindness that affects women in particular.

4. A fair start for all girls is critical for the health of women

Many of the health problems faced by adult women have their origins in childhood

Proper nutrition is a key determinant of health, both in childhood and beyond. The nutritional status of girls is particularly important due to their future potential reproductive role and the intergenerational repercussions of poor female nutrition. Preventing child abuse and neglect and ensuring a supportive environment in early childhood will help children to achieve optimal physical, social and emotional development. These will also help avoid risky behaviours and a significant burden of disease, including mental health disorders and substance use later in life.

Changing behaviour now brings major health benefits later

It is essential to address the health and development needs of adolescents if they are to make a healthy transition to adulthood. Societies must tackle the factors that promote potentially harmful behaviours in relation to sex, tobacco and alcohol use, diet and physical activity, as well as provide adolescents with the support they need to avoid these harmful behaviours. In many high-income countries, adolescent girls are increasingly using alcohol and tobacco, and obesity is on the rise. Supporting adolescents to establish healthy habits in adolescence will bring major health benefits later in life, including reduced mortality and disability due to cardiovascular diseases, stroke and cancers.

Addressing the needs of older women will be a major challenge to health systems

Because they tend to live longer than men, women represent a growing proportion of all older people. Societies need to prepare now to prevent and manage the chronic health problems often associated with old age. Establishing healthy habits at younger ages can help women to live active and healthy lives until well into old age. Societies must also prepare for the costs associated with the care of older women. Many high-income countries currently direct large proportions of their social and health budgets to care for the elderly. In low-income settings, such care is often the responsibility of the family, usually of its female members. Policies are needed in relation to health financing, pension and tax reform, access to formal employment and associated pension and social protection, and to the provision of residential and community care.

5. Societies and their health systems are failing women

Health system shortfalls deprive women of health care

The reasons why health systems fail women are often complex and related to the biases they face in society. However, these shortfalls can be understood and they can and should be challenged and changed. For example, women face higher health costs than men due to their greater use of health care yet they are more likely than their male counterparts to be poor, unemployed or else engaged in part-time work or work in the informal sector that offers no health benefits. One of the keys to improving women's health therefore, is the removal of financial barriers to health care. For instance, where there are user fees for maternal health services, households pay a substantial proportion of the cost of facility-based services, and the expense of complicated deliveries is often catastrophic. Evidence from several countries shows that removing user fees for maternal health care, especially for deliveries, can both stimulate demand and lead to increased uptake of essential services. Removing financial barriers to care must be accompanied by efforts to ensure that health services are appropriate, acceptable, of high quality and responsive to the needs of girls and women.

Health systems depend on women as providers of health care

Paradoxically, health systems are often unresponsive to the needs of women despite the fact that women themselves are major contributors to health, through their roles as primary caregivers in the family and also as health-care providers in both the formal and informal health sectors. The backbone of the health system, women are nevertheless rarely represented in executive or management-level positions, tending to be concentrated in lower-paid jobs and exposed to greater occupational health risks. In their roles as informal health-care providers at home or the community, women are often unsupported, unrecognized and unremunerated.

Societal failings damage women's health

Women's health is profoundly affected by the ways in which they are treated and the status they are given by society as a whole. Where women continue to be discriminated against or subjected to violence, their health suffers. Where they are excluded by law from the ownership of land or property or from the right to divorce, their social and physical vulnerability is increased. At its most extreme, social or cultural gender bias can lead to violent death or female infanticide. Even where progress is being made there are reasons to keep pushing for more. While there has been much progress in girls' access to education for example, there is still a male–female gap when it comes to secondary education, access to employment and equal pay. Meanwhile, the greater economic independence enjoyed by some women as a result of more widespread female employment may have benefits for health, but globally, women are less well protected in the workplace, both in terms of security and working conditions.

Developing a shared agenda for women's health

In publishing this report WHO seeks to identify key areas for reform, both within the health sector and beyond. Primary health care, with its focus on equity, solidarity and social justice, offers an opportunity to make a difference, through policy action in the following four areas.

Building strong leadership and a coherent institutional response

National and international responses to women's health issues tend to be fragmented and limited in scope. Identifying mechanisms to foster bold, participatory leadership around a clear and coherent agenda for action will be critical to making progress. The involvement and full participation of women and women's organizations is essential. The significant advances in women's health achieved in some countries indicate that it can be done. The interventions are known and the resources are attainable.

The Millennium Development Goals (MDGs) have been vitally important in maintaining a focus on development and in setting benchmarks in the face of many competing claims on the world's attention. The existence of a separate goal on maternal health draws attention to the lack of progress in this area, and has attracted both political and financial support for accelerating change. The addition of the target on universal access to reproductive health has helped broaden the scope of the goal. There is now a need to extend attention to the many other challenges to and determinants of women's health described in this report. In doing so, attention should be paid to ensuring gender equality and women's empowerment (MDG3). The situation is complex due to the way women's issues are handled both within and between governments and international organizations, with multiple initiatives competing for resources. More collaboration is needed to develop supportive structures, incentives and accountability mechanisms for improving women's health.

Making health systems work for women

The report highlights the need to strengthen health systems so that they are better geared to meet women's needs – in terms of access, comprehensiveness and responsiveness. This is not just an issue in relation to sexual and reproductive health – it is relevant throughout the life-course. Progress in increasing access to the services that could make a difference to women's health is patchy and uneven. Some services, such as antenatal care, are more likely to be in place than others, such as those related to mental health, sexual violence and cervical cancer screening and care. Abysmally low levels of coverage with basic interventions, such as immunization and skilled birth attendance, are found in several countries, and not only in those with humanitarian crises. Exclusion from health care of those in need, particularly the poor and vulnerable, is common, and the equity gap is increasing in many countries. Approaches to extending coverage must deal with the content of benefit packages and must include a greater range of services for girls and women of all ages. They must also address the issue of financial protection, by moving away from user charges and promoting prepayment and pooling schemes.

Healthier societies: leveraging changes in public policy

The report shows how social and economic determinants of health impact on women. Many of the main causes of women's morbidity and mortality – in both rich and poor countries – have their origins in societies' attitudes to women, which are reflected in the structures and systems that set policies, determine services and create opportunities. While technical solutions can mitigate immediate consequences, sustainable progress will depend on more fundamental change. Public policies have the potential to influence exposure to risks, access to care and the consequences of ill-health in women and girls. The report provides examples of such policies – from targeted action to encourage girls to enrol in school and pursue their education (by ensuring a safe school environment and promoting later marriage), to measures to build "age-friendly" environments and increase opportunities for older women to contribute productively to society. Intersectoral collaboration is required to identify and promote actions outside the health sector that can enhance health outcomes for women. Broader strategies, such as poverty reduction, increased access to literacy, training and education, and increased opportunities for women to participate in economic activities, will also contribute to making sustainable progress in women's health. Experience suggests that this requires a gender equality and rights-based approach that harnesses the energy of civil society and recognizes the need for political engagement.

Building the knowledge base and monitoring progress

The report highlights major gaps in knowledge that seriously limit what we can say with real authority about the health of women in different parts of the world. While much is known about women's health, many gaps remain in our understanding of the dimensions and nature of the special challenges they face and how these can be effectively addressed. We must also be able to measure progress – and we must do it now. The foundations of better information about women and health need to be strengthened, starting with civil registration systems that generate vital statistics – including cause of death by age and by sex – and collection and use of age- and sex-disaggregated data on common problems. These data are essential for programme planning and management and without such systems, efforts to monitor changes in, for example, maternal mortality will remain thwarted. Research must systematically incorporate attention to sex and gender in design, analysis and interpretation of findings. We must focus more attention on assessing progress in increasing coverage with key interventions, together with the tracking of relevant policies, health system performance measures and equity patterns.

Conclusion

In reviewing the evidence and setting an agenda for the future, this report points the way towards the actions needed to better the health of girls and women around the world. The report aims to inform policy dialogue and stimulate action by countries, agencies and development partners.

While this report highlights differences between women and men, it is not a report just about women and not a report just for women. Addressing women's health is a necessary and effective approach to strengthening health systems overall – action that will benefit everyone. Improving women's health matters to women, to their families, communities and societies at large.

Improve women's health – improve the world.

CHAPTER 1

UNDERSTANDING WOMEN'S HEALTH IN THE WORLD TODAY

Figure 1 **Mortality and disease burden (DALYs) in females by region, age group and broad causes, 2004**

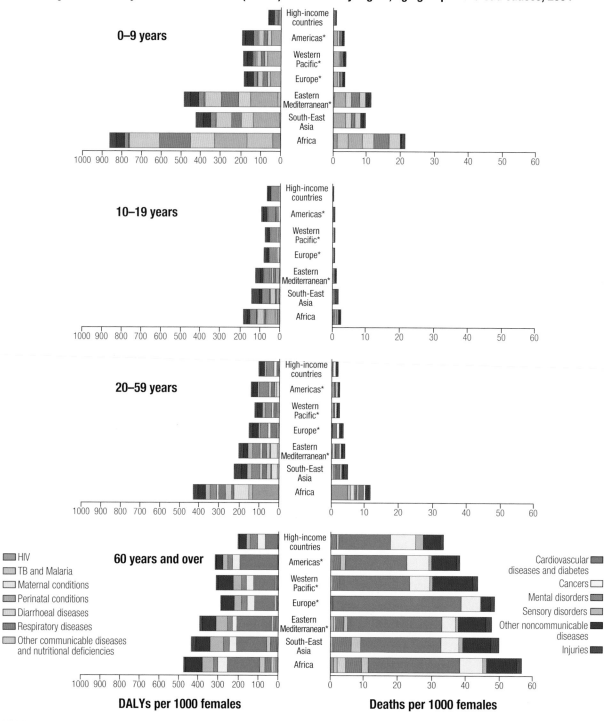

DALYs per 1000 females   Deaths per 1000 females

* High-income countries are excluded from the regional groups.
Source: World Health Organization.[1]

Why focus on women and health? The response, as described in this report, is that women and girls have particular health needs and that health systems are failing them.

What are these needs? There are conditions that only women experience and that have negative health impacts that only women suffer. Some of these conditions, such as pregnancy and childbirth, are not in themselves diseases, but normal physiological and social processes that carry health risks and require health care.

Some health challenges affect both women and men but, because they have a greater or different impact on women, they require responses that are tailored specifically to women's needs. Other conditions affect men and women more or less equally, but women face greater difficulties in getting the health care they need. Furthermore, gender-based inequalities – as in education, income and employment – limit the ability of women to protect their health and achieve optimal health status.

Women's health matters not only to women themselves. It is also crucial to the health of the children they will bear. This underlines an important point: paying due attention to the health of girls and women today is an investment not just for the present but also for future generations. This implies addressing the underlying social and economic determinants of women's health – including education, which directly benefits women and is important for the survival, growth and development of their children. We return to this issue later in this chapter and in Chapter 7.

Analyses of women's health often focus on, or are limited to, specific periods of women's lives (the reproductive ages, for instance) or specific health challenges such as the human immunodeficiency virus (HIV), maternal health, violence, or mental ill-health. This report, by contrast, provides data on women's health throughout the life course and covers the full range of causes of death and disability in the major world regions.

The report is based on data currently available to WHO. However, the analysis reveals serious shortcomings in the systems needed to generate timely and reliable data on the major health challenges that girls and women face, especially in low-income countries. Many of the conclusions are based on extrapolation from incomplete data. Nonetheless, the available information points clearly to challenges and health concerns that must be addressed urgently if girls and women are to realize fully their human right to health and, by extension, to their economic and social rights.

The aim of the detailed epidemiological analysis in the following chapters is to provide the foundation for a comprehensive understanding of the health challenges faced by girls and women around the world throughout their lives. From this overview of the burden of ill-health women face at different ages – not only deaths but also non-fatal, often chronic conditions – four main themes emerge (Figure 1). These are explored more fully in later chapters.

Box 1   Burden of disease and DALYs

Diseases that cause a large number of deaths are clear public health priorities. However, mortality statistics alone do not show the loss of health among girls and women caused by chronic diseases, injuries, sensory disorders and mental disorders. Disability-adjusted life years (DALYs) incorporate lost healthy years of life due to premature mortality and to non-fatal chronic conditions into measures of disease burden in populations,[1] and give greater weight to deaths that occur at younger ages. The DALY extends the concept of potential years of life lost due to premature death to include equivalent years of healthy life lost by virtue of being in a state of poor health or disability. One DALY can be thought of as one lost year of healthy life, and the burden of disease can be thought of as a measurement of the gap between current health status and an ideal situation where everyone lives into old age, free from disease and disability.

First, the leading global causes of the overall burden of disease in females are lower respiratory infections, depression and diarrhoeal diseases. Box 1 explains how the burden of disease in females is calculated in disability-adjusted life years, or DALYs. Neuropsychiatric conditions and sensory disorders – related, for example, to vision and hearing – are also important causes of DALYs worldwide. Infectious diseases continue to cause over half the DALYs in the African Region but have a much smaller impact in other regions.[1]

Second, in all regions and age groups, girls and women in higher income countries have lower levels of mortality and burden of disease than those who live in lower income countries. Across all ages, the highest mortality and disability rates are found in Africa.

Third, the causes of death and disability among girls and women vary throughout the life course. In childhood, most deaths and disabilities result from communicable diseases such as HIV, diarrhoeal and respiratory diseases, malaria, and maternal and perinatal conditions. At older ages, patterns of death and disability change to noncommunicable chronic diseases such as heart disease, stroke and cancers. The single exception is in Africa, where communicable diseases remain the chief causes of female deaths up to the age of 60 years.

Fourth, there are significant regional variations in the composition of the overall burden of death and disability. In Africa and South-East Asia, communicable diseases are important causes of death and disability at all ages. However, in women aged 60 years and over, in all regions, most deaths are due to noncommunicable diseases.

The following chapters explore the varying patterns of death and disability more fully and identify policy and programme implications that emerge from the data. This initial chapter gives an overall summary of the health status of girls and women, describes critical factors that influence their health – including gender-based inequities and economic and social factors – and shows that women are not simply potential consumers of health care but are also critical for the provision of care in both the formal and informal sectors.

Women around the world

Most of the world's women live in low- or middle-income countries, almost half of them in the South-East Asia and Western Pacific regions. Only 15% of the world's 3.3 billion females live in high-income countries (Table 1). More than one female in every three lives in a low-income country. Since low-income countries tend to have younger populations than high-income countries, one in every two children under nine years of age lives in a low-income country. By contrast, one in three women aged 60 years or more lives in a high-income country. High-income countries have the largest proportions of population aged 60 years or more (Figure 2).

Table 1 **Number and distribution of the world's women and girls by age group and country income group, 2007**

	Low-income countries		Middle-income countries		High-income countries		Global total
Age group	000s	%	000s	%	000s	%	000s
0–9	300 768	50	241 317	40	57 456	10	599 541
10–19	267 935	45	263 464	44	61 577	10	592 975
20–59	580 014	34	875 052	51	276 140	16	1 731 206
60+	86 171	22	183 099	48	115 681	30	384 952
Total	1 234 888	37	1 562 932	47	510 854	15	3 308 673

Source: United Nations Population Division.[2]

The regions with the largest proportion of children and young people under the age of 20 years are Africa and South-East Asia.

Today the lives of females of all ages and in all countries are being shaped by a series of factors – epidemiological, demographic, social, cultural, economic and environmental. These same factors influence the lives of males but some adversities affect girls and women in particular. For example, it is a natural biological phenomenon that sex ratios at birth tend slightly to favour boys. Thus, for every 100 boys born there are between 94 (Africa) to 98 (other parts of the world) girls. However, in some settings, societal discrimination against females and parental preference for sons result in skewed sex ratios. In India, for instance, the 2001 census recorded only 93 girls per 100 boys – a sharp decline from 1961 when the number of girls was nearly 98. In some parts of India, there are fewer than 80 girls for every 100 boys. Low sex ratios have also been recorded in other Asian countries – most notably China where, according to a survey in 2005, only 84 girls were born for every 100 boys. This was slightly up from 81 during 2001–2004, but much lower than 93 girls per 100 boys as shown among children born in the late 1980s.[3]

Increasing life expectancy

Females generally live longer than males – on average by six to eight years. This difference is partly due to an inherent biological advantage for the female. But it also reflects behavioural differences between men and women. As Chapter 2 shows, newborn girls are more likely to survive to their first birthday than newborn boys are.[4] This advantage continues throughout life: women tend to have lower rates of mortality at all ages, probably due to a combination of the genetic and behavioural factors that are described in the chapters that follow.[1] Women's longevity advantage becomes most apparent in old age, and this is explored more fully in Chapter 6. This may be the result of lower lifetime risk behaviours such as smoking and alcohol use. Alternatively, it may be the effect of harder-to-identify biological advantages that result in relatively lower rates of cardiovascular disease and cancer in women. The gap in life expectancy between women and men is narrowing to some extent in some developed countries. This may be due to increased smoking among women and falling rates of cardiovascular disease among men, but the question is open to debate.[5,6]

The female advantage in life expectancy may be a relatively recent phenomenon. Accurate historical data are hard to come by, but there is evidence that in 17th century England and Wales the life expectancy of men surpassed that of women.[7,8] Part of the explanation may lie in the low social position of women at the time, coupled with high rates of mortality that were often associated with pregnancy and childbearing.

Globally, female life expectancy at birth has increased by nearly 20 years since the early 1950s when it was just 51 years (Figure 3). In 2007, female life expectancy at birth was 70 years compared with 65 years

Figure 2 **Distribution of women by major age group and region, 2007**

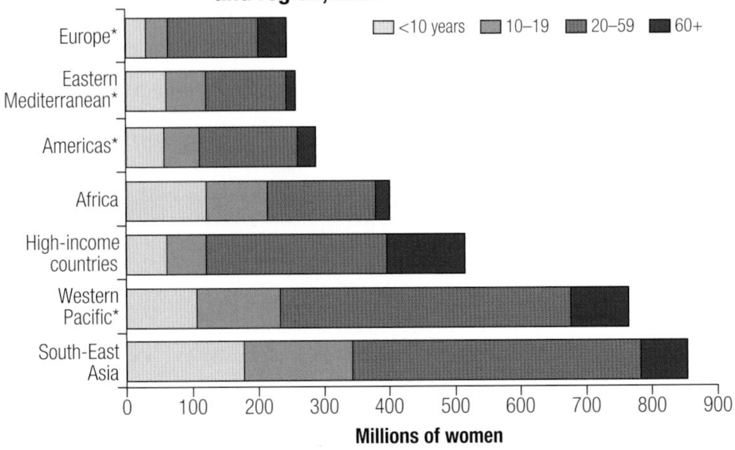

*High-income countries are excluded from the regional groups.
Source: United Nations Population Division.[2]

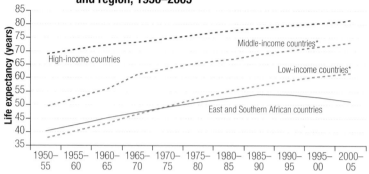

Figure 3 **Female life expectancy at birth by country income group and region, 1950–2005**

* Excluding East and Southern African countries.

Source: United Nations Population Division.[2]

for males. Life expectancy for women is now more than 80 years in at least 35 countries, but the picture is not uniformly positive. For instance, life expectancy at birth for women in the African Region was estimated at only 54 years in 2007 – the lowest of any region. In some African countries, particularly in East and Southern Africa, the lack of improvement in life expectancy is mainly due to HIV/AIDS and maternal mortality, but these are not the only factors at work. In a few countries, women's life expectancy is equal to or shorter than men's as a result of the social disadvantages that women face.[4]

However, life expectancy alone tells only part of the story; the extra years of life for women are not always lived in good health. In low-income countries especially, the difference between women and men in terms of healthy life expectancy is marginal (only one year) and in several countries, healthy life expectancy for women is lower than for men.[4]

The health transition

One of the most striking features of recent decades has been a shift in the underlying causes of death and disease around the world. This so-called "health transition" affects men, women and children in all countries and stems from changes in three interrelated and mutually reinforcing elements – demographic structures, patterns of disease and risk factors.

The *demographic* transition is characterized by lower mortality rates among children under five years and declining fertility rates, which result in an ageing population. The average number of children per woman has fallen globally from 4.3 during the early 1970s to 2.6 by 2005–2010 (Table 2). These declines are largely the result of increasing use of contraception (see Chapter 4).

The *epidemiological* transition reflects a shift in the main causes of death and disease away from infectious diseases, such as diarrhoea and pneumonia (diseases traditionally associated with poorer countries), towards noncommunicable diseases such as cardiovascular disease, stroke and cancers (long considered to be the burden of richer countries).

The *risk* transition is characterized by a reduction in risk factors for infectious diseases (undernutrition, unsafe water and poor sanitation, for example) and an increase in risk factors for chronic diseases (such as overweight, and use of alcohol and tobacco).

This health transition is occurring at different rates in different countries. In many middle-income countries, including much of Latin America and China,

Table 2 **Total fertility (average number of children per woman) by major region, 1970–2005**

Area	1970–75	2005–2010
World	4.32	2.56
Africa	6.69	4.61
Asia	4.76	2.35
Europe	2.19	1.50
Latin America and the Caribbean	5.01	2.26
North America	2.07	2.04
Oceania	3.29	2.44

Source: United Nations Population Division.[2]

the health transition is already quite pronounced. In Mexico in 2006, for instance, only 13% of deaths (both male and female) were caused by communicable, nutritional and maternal factors compared with over 60% in 1955. Even though death rates due to noncommunicable diseases have declined in Mexico, these diseases cause an increasing proportion of total deaths, reaching 80% by 2006 (Figure 4). As in many other countries, in Mexico women were less likely to die from injuries than men were. During the 1980s, 23% of male deaths were caused by injuries, but only 7% of women died from injuries. The health transition is least advanced in Africa, where patterns of mortality among girls and women are still characterized by a predominance of infectious diseases (Figure 5).

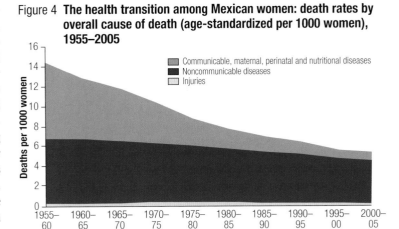

Figure 4 **The health transition among Mexican women: death rates by overall cause of death (age-standardized per 1000 women), 1955–2005**

Sources: World Health Organization.[9] United Nations Population Division.[2]

In the early stages of the health transition, women and children face high levels of mortality, often linked to nutritional deficiencies, unsafe water and sanitation, smoke from solid fuels used for cooking and heating, and lack of care during childhood, pregnancy and childbearing. These traditional risks not only exact a direct toll on the health of women and children but also have an adverse impact on the health of the next generation. Women with poor nutrition, infectious diseases and inadequate access to care tend to have infants with low birth weight whose chances of health and survival are compromised.[10,11] Public health interventions have long focused on combating these problems through improved nutrition, cleaner household

Figure 5 **Women's deaths from communicable, maternal, perinatal and nutritional conditions as a percentage of total women's deaths, 2004**

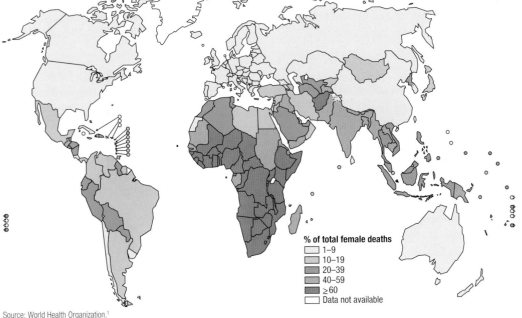

% of total female deaths
- 1–9
- 10–19
- 20–39
- 40–59
- ≥60
- Data not available

Source: World Health Organization.[1]

environments, and better health care. However, new or previously unrecognized health challenges continue to emerge – including overweight and obesity, lack of exercise, use of tobacco and alcohol, violence against women, and environmental risks such as poor urban air quality and adverse climate change. The impact of these emerging risks varies at different levels of socioeconomic development. Urban air pollution, for example, is often a greater risk to health in middle-income countries compared with high-income countries because the latter have made greater progress in environmental and public health policies.

The risk transition reflects differences in the patterns of behaviour of men and women. For example, in many settings, use of tobacco and alcohol was traditionally higher among men than women. More recently, however, smoking rates among females have started to approach those of males; the health consequences (e.g. increased rates of cardiovascular diseases and cancers) will emerge in the future. In low-income and middle-income countries, alcohol use is generally higher among men. However, in many higher income countries, male and female patterns of alcohol use are beginning to converge.

Socioeconomic inequalities adversely affect health

Socioeconomic status is a major determinant of health for both sexes. As a general rule, women in high-income countries live longer and are less likely to suffer from ill-health than women in low-income countries. In high-income countries, death rates among children and younger women are very low and most deaths occur after the age of 60 years (Figure 6). In low-income countries the picture is quite different. The population is younger and death rates at young ages are higher, with most deaths occurring among girls, adolescents and younger adult women.

In high-income countries, noncommunicable diseases, such as heart disease, stroke, dementias and cancers, predominate in the 10 leading causes of death, accounting for more than four in every 10 female deaths. By contrast, in low-income countries, maternal and perinatal conditions and communicable diseases (e.g. lower respiratory infections, diarrhoeal diseases and HIV/AIDS) are prominent and account for over 38% of total female deaths (Table 3).

Figure 6 **Female deaths by age group and country income group, 2007**

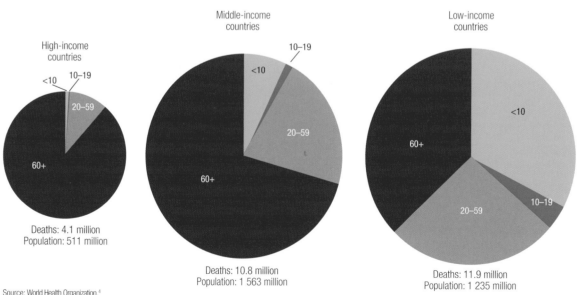

Source: World Health Organization.[4]

Poverty and low socioeconomic status are associated with worse health outcomes. Data from 66 developing countries show that child mortality rates among the poorest 20% of households are almost double those in the richest 20%.[4] In both high-income and low-income countries, levels of maternal mortality may be up to three times higher among disadvantaged ethnic groups than among other women.[12,13] There are similar differentials in terms of use of health-care services. For instance, women in the poorest households are least likely to have a skilled birth attendant with them during childbirth (see below).

Gender inequities affect women's health

The adverse impact on health of low socioeconomic status is compounded for women by gender inequities. In many countries and societies, women and girls are treated as socially inferior. Behavioural and other social norms, codes of conduct and laws perpetuate the subjugation of females and condone violence against them. Unequal power relations and gendered norms and values translate into differential access to and control over health resources, both within

Table 3 **Ten leading causes of death in females by country income group, 2004**

Rank	Cause (World)	Deaths (000s)	%		Rank	Cause (Low-income countries)	Deaths (000s)	%
1	Ischaemic heart disease	3371	12.2		1	Lower respiratory infections	1397	11.4
2	Stroke	3051	11.1		2	Ischaemic heart disease	1061	8.7
3	Lower respiratory infections	2014	7.3		3	Diarrhoeal diseases	851	7.0
4	COPD*	1405	5.1		4	Stroke	749	6.1
5	Diarrhoeal diseases	1037	3.8		5	HIV/AIDS	742	6.1
6	HIV/AIDS	1013	3.7		6	Maternal conditions	442	3.6
7	Diabetes mellitus	633	2.3		7	Neonatal infections**	426	3.5
8	Prematurity and low birth weight	567	2.1		8	Prematurity and low birth weight	405	3.3
9	Neonatal infections**	546	2.0		9	Malaria	404	3.3
10	Hypertensive heart disease	530	1.9		10	COPD*	404	3.3

Rank	Cause (Middle-income countries)	Deaths (000s)	%		Rank	Cause (High-income countries)	Deaths (000s)	%
1	Stroke	1842	16.4		1	Ischaemic heart disease	650	15.8
2	Ischaemic heart disease	1659	14.8		2	Stroke	459	11.2
3	COPD*	875	7.8		3	Alzheimer and other dementias	195	4.7
4	Lower respiratory infections	451	4.0		4	Lower respiratory infections	165	4.0
5	Hypertensive heart disease	319	2.8		5	Breast cancer	163	4.0
6	Diabetes mellitus	309	2.8		6	Trachea, bronchus and lung cancers	159	3.9
7	HIV/AIDS	264	2.4		7	Colon and rectum cancers	130	3.2
8	Breast cancer	231	2.1		8	COPD*	126	3.1
9	Stomach cancer	201	1.8		9	Diabetes mellitus	123	3.0
10	Trachea, bronchus and lung cancers	191	1.7		10	Hypertensive heart disease	91	2.2

*Chronic obstructive pulmonary disease.
**Includes severe neonatal infections and other non-infectious causes arising in the perinatal period.
Source: World Health Organization.[1]

families and beyond. Gender inequalities in the allocation of resources, such as income, education, health care, nutrition and political voice, are strongly associated with poor health and reduced well-being. Thus, across a range of health problems, girls and women face differential exposures and vulnerabilities that are often poorly recognized.

Although women's political participation is growing, men still wield political control in most societies and, by extension, they wield social and economic control as well.[14] No reliable data are available on the proportion of women living in poverty, but women are particularly vulnerable to income poverty because they are less likely than men to be in formal employment and much of their labour is unpaid.[15] In many developing countries, a large proportion of agricultural workers are women and many are unpaid as this is part of their role within the family.[15]

Women's participation in paid, non-agricultural employment has increased since 1990 so that by 2005 almost 40% of employees were women.[14] Nonetheless, employment ratios (i.e. the number of employed persons as a percentage of the population of working age) are significantly higher for men than for women, with a gender gap that ranges from 15% in developed regions to more than 40% in South Asia and in the Middle East and North Africa.[16] Even when they are in formal employment, women generally earn less than men. The ratio of female-to-male earned income is well below parity in all countries for which data are available.[17]

Because they are less likely to be part of the formal labour market, women lack access to job security and the benefits of social protection, including access to health care. Within the formal workforce, women often face challenges related to their lower status,[18] suffer discrimination and sexual harassment,[19] and have to balance the demands of paid work and work at home, giving rise to work-related fatigue, infections, mental ill-health and other problems.[20]

Data from nearly 50 national Demographic and Health Surveys show that on average a woman is head of one in five households and that these households are particularly vulnerable to poverty.[21] Nor is the problem confined to developing countries. According to the United States Census Bureau, more than 28% of women and children in female-headed households live below the federal poverty line compared with less than 14% of families in male-headed households and 5% of married-couple families.[22]

Women's health may also be at risk as a result of their traditional family responsibilities. For instance, women prepare most of the family food and, where solid fuels are used for cooking, girls and women often suffer as a result of exposure to indoor air pollution. Breathing air tainted by the burning of solid fuels is estimated to be responsible for 641 000 of the 1.3 million deaths worldwide due to chronic obstructive pulmonary disorder (COPD) among women each year.[1] The burden of COPD caused by exposure to indoor smoke is over 50% higher among women than among men.

Figure 7 **Distribution of those who usually collect water in 35 developing countries, 2005–2006**

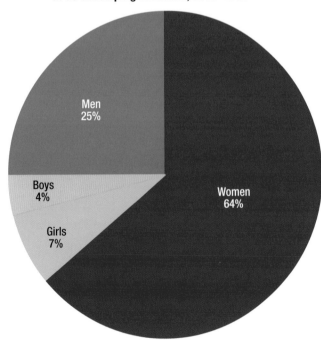

Source: UNICEF and the World Health Organization.[23]

Women are disproportionately responsible for collecting household fuel and water (Figure 7).[23] The time spent on collecting household fuel and water could otherwise be spent on income-generation, education, or care for family members, all of which are related to the health status of women and of their families.

Achieving parity in education – in primary school and beyond – is critical if women are to engage fully in society and the economy. Female education not only directly benefits women themselves but is also important for the survival, growth and development of their children. In all countries with relevant data, child mortality rates are highest in households where the education of the mother is lowest.[4] Despite impressive gains in female enrolment in primary education between 2000 and 2006, girls still account for 55% of the out-of-school population. Over 580 million women are illiterate (twice the number of illiterate men) and more than 70 million girls are not in school.[24]

In some settings, gender inequity is associated with particular forms of violence against females – including violence by an intimate partner, sexual violence by acquaintances and strangers, child sexual abuse, forced sexual initiation, and female genital mutilation. Women and girls are also vulnerable to less well-documented forms of abuse or exploitation, such as human trafficking or "honour killings" for perceived transgressions of their social role. These acts are associated with a wide range of health problems in women such as injuries, unwanted pregnancies, abortions, depression, anxiety and eating disorders, substance use, sexually transmitted infections and, of course, premature death.[25,26]

Women amid conflicts and crisis

Women face particular problems in disasters and emergencies. Available data suggest that there is a pattern of gender differentiation at all stages of a disaster: exposure to risk, risk perception, preparedness, response, physical impact, psychological impact, recovery and reconstruction.[27] Studies of several recent disasters in South-East Asia found that more women than men died as a result of the disaster.[28] In situations of conflict and crisis, women are often at greater risk of sexual coercion and rape.[29] In the midst of natural disasters and armed conflicts, access to health services may be even more restricted than normal, contributing to physical and mental health problems that include unwanted pregnancy, and maternal and perinatal mortality. Even when health care is available, women may be unable to access it because of cultural restrictions or their household responsibilities.[30]

Women and the health-care system

The socioeconomic and gender-based inequalities that women face are played out in their access to and use of health-care services. As already noted, and as highlighted in the chapters that follow, the poorest women are generally least likely to use health-care services. The reasons are complex: services may be unavailable or inaccessible, or women may be unable to find affordable transport. Sociocultural norms also often limit women's mobility and interaction with male health providers.

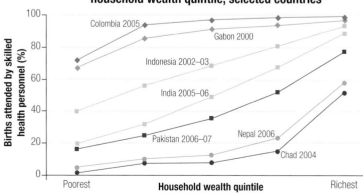

Figure 8 **Births attended by skilled health personnel, by household wealth quintile, selected countries**

Source: Demographic and Health Surveys in selected countries, 2000–2007.

The way that socioeconomic inequality plays out in different settings is important for determining the most effective policy and programme responses. In some settings, barriers to access to health care affect all households except the wealthiest (Figure 8). In Chad and Nepal, for instance, only the wealthiest households use a skilled birth attendant at delivery. In India, Indonesia and Pakistan, while access to health services is better across all income groups, the wealthiest benefit most and poorer households are left behind. In Colombia and Gabon, the use of skilled birth personnel is relatively high across most income groups but not in the poorest group. These different patterns of inequality imply the need for different programmatic interventions that range from targeting the poorest to strengthening the whole health system, to a combination of both strategies.[31]

It is a paradox that health services are so often inaccessible to women or unresponsive to their needs given that health systems are so highly dependent on women. Women are the main providers of care within the family and constitute the backbone both of the formal health workforce and of informal health-care provision. Women predominate in the formal health workforce in many countries (Figure 9). The available data are of variable quality and derive from different sources but they indicate overall that women make up over 50% of formal health-care workers in many countries.[34,35] With an estimated 59 million health workers in full-time employment around the world,[36] this suggests that some 30 million of them are women. Many millions more women are informal providers of health care.

Women tend to be concentrated in occupations that may be considered to have lower status – such as nursing, midwifery, and community health services – and are a minority among the highly trained professionals.[35] Nursing, midwifery, the community health workforce and other front-line providers remain predominantly female almost everywhere while men continue to dominate among doctors and dentists. Notable exceptions exist, however. For example, Estonia, Mongolia, the Russian Federation and Sudan report more female than male doctors.

Typically, more than 70% of doctors are male while more than 70% of nurses are female – a marked gender imbalance. In many countries, female health-service providers are particularly scarce in rural areas, a situation that may arise in part because it is unsafe for females to live alone in some isolated areas. The picture may well be different if traditional birth attendants and village volunteers were included in the calculations as these are the domains of women in many countries. However, this information is rarely routinely available. Moreover, there are some notable exceptions. For example, Ethiopia and Pakistan are among the countries that have sought actively to recruit and train female health workers in rural areas.

Figure 9 **Share of women in the health workforce, selected countries, 1989–1997**

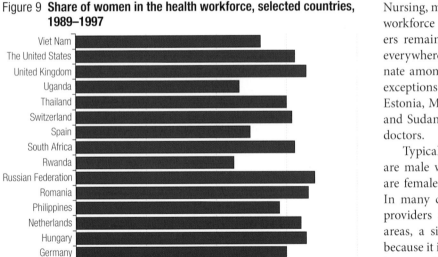

Sources: Gupta N et al.[32] Lavallée R, Hanvoravongchai P, Gupta N.[33]

Female health workers face several work-related health problems. Because there are more women in the health-care workforce and because female health-care workers are often working with sharps, women account for about two-thirds of all global hepatitis B and C infections and HIV infections due to needlestick injuries.[37] Women are also prone to musculoskeletal injuries (caused by lifting) and burn-out.[37–41] Female health workers are exposed to hazardous drugs that are mutagenic and possibly carcinogenic, and to chemical hazards such as disinfectants and sterilants which cause asthma,[42] as well as to adverse reproductive outcomes such as spontaneous abortion and congenital malformations. Female community health workers may also be subjected to violence.[34]

Conclusion

This introductory chapter has summarized some of the health challenges faced by women across their lives and has given an overview of some of the underlying determinants of women's health. It is clear that women around the world face health challenges at every stage of their lives from early childhood to old age, and whether at home, at work or in wider society. The chapters that follow look in greater detail at these challenges as they manifest at different stages of life and show how health systems are failing to respond adequately to women's needs.

Summary findings and implications

■ There have been major improvements in life expectancy among women over the past half-century but not all women have benefited. Thus, there remain significant variations in life expectancy and health for women in different parts of the world. A woman born in a high-income country can expect to live for more than 80 years; by contrast, a woman born in East or Southern Africa can expect to live only for 50 years.

■ A health transition is sweeping around the world, leading to a shift in the patterns of death and disease – away from infectious diseases and maternal conditions to noncommunicable and chronic diseases. However, the transition is happening at different rates in different parts of the world. In many settings women are confronted by a dual burden of traditional health threats related to infectious diseases and maternal conditions alongside emerging challenges associated with noncommunicable chronic diseases.

■ Women provide the bulk of health care worldwide, both in the formal health-care setting as well as in the informal sector and in the home. Yet women's own needs for health care are often poorly addressed, especially among rural and poor communities.

■ Both sex and gender have a significant impact on the health of women and must be considered when developing appropriate strategies for health promotion and for the prevention and treatment of ill-health. Gender inequality, both alone and in combination with biological differences, can increase women's vulnerability or exposure to certain risks: it may lead to differences which are not always recognized in the manifestation, severity and consequences of disease, or to different responses by the health services, or different consequences, and it may limit women's access to resources and to health-care information and services.

■ Societies and their health systems need to be better geared to meet women's health needs in terms of access, comprehensiveness and responsiveness. Policies and programmes must ensure that gender norms and socioeconomic inequalities do not limit women's ability to access health information and health-care services. Broader strategies such as poverty reduction, increased literacy, training and education, and increased opportunities for participation in economic, social and political activities will contribute to progress in women's health.

References

1. *The global burden of disease: 2004 update*. Geneva, World Health Organization, 2008.
2. *World population prospects: the 2006 revision*. New York, NY, United Nations Population Division, 2007.
3. Zhu WX, Lu L, Hesketh T. China's excess males, sex selective abortion and one child policy: analysis of data from 2005 national intercensus survey. *BMJ (Clinical Research Ed.)*, 2009, 338:b1211. PMID:19359290 doi:10.1136/bmj.b1211
4. *World health statistics 2009*. Geneva, World Health Organization, 2009.
5. Meslé F. Ecart d'espérance de vie entre les sexes: les raisons du recul de l'avantage féminin. *Revue d'Epidemiologie et de Sante Publique*, 2004, 52:333–352. PMID:15480291 doi:10.1016/S0398-7620(04)99063-3
6. Glei DA, Horiuchi S. The narrowing sex differential in life expectancy in high-income populations: effects of differences in the age pattern of mortality. *Population Studies*, 2007, 61:141–159. PMID:17558883 doi:10.1080/00324720701331433
7. Wrigley EA, Davies RS, Oeppen JE, Schofield RS. *English population history from family reconstitution, 1580–1837*. New York, NY, Cambridge University Press, 1997.
8. Vallin J. Mortalité, sexe et genre. In: Caselli G, Wunsch G, Vallin J, eds. *Démographie: analyse et synthèse. III. Les déterminants de la mortalité*. Paris, Institut national d'études démographiques (INED), 2002.
9. WHO mortality database. Geneva, March 2009 (http://www.who.int/healthinfo/morttables/en/index.html).
10. Berkman DS et al. Effects of stunting, diarrhoeal disease, and parasitic infection during infancy on cognition in late childhood: a follow-up study. *Lancet*, 2002, 359:564–571. PMID:11867110 doi:10.1016/S0140-6736(02)07744-9
11. Mendez MA, Adair LS. Severity and timing of stunting in the first two years of life affect performance on cognitive tests in late childhood. *The Journal of Nutrition*, 1999, 129:1555–1562. PMID:10419990
12. *Australia's health 2008*. Canberra, Australian Institute of Health and Welfare, 2008.
13. Anachebe NF. Racial and ethnic disparities in infant and maternal mortality. *Ethnicity & Disease*, 2006, 16 suppl 3;71–76. PMID:16774028
14. *The Millennium Development Goals report 2007*. New York, NY, United Nations, 2007 (http://www.un.org/millenniumgoals/pdf/mdg2007.pdf, accessed 18 July 2009).
15. *World development indicators 2008*. Washington, DC, The World Bank, 2008.
16. *MDGs and gender*. New York, NY, United Nations Development Fund for Women, 2008 (http://www.unifem.org/progress/2008/mdgsGender_2.html, accessed 20 April 2009).
17. *Human development report 2007/2008*. New York, NY, United Nations Development Programme, 2008.
18. Hall E. Gender, work control and stress: a theoretical discussion and an empirical test. *International Journal of Health Services*, 1989, 19:725–745. PMID:2583884 doi:10.2190/5MYW-PGP9-4M72-TPXF
19. Paoli P, Merllié D. *Third European survey on working conditions 2000*. Dublin, European Foundation for the Improvement of Living and Working Conditions, 2001.
20. Östlin P. Gender inequalities in health: the significance of work. In: Wamala S, Lynch J, eds. *Gender and socioeconomic inequalities in health*. Lund, Studentlitteratur, 2002.
21. Mukuria A, Alboulafia C, Themme A. *The context of women's health: results from the Demographic and Health Surveys, 1994–2001*. DHS Comparative Reports No.11. Calverton, MD, ORC Macro, 2005.
22. *Summarizing the new US Census Bureau report on Income and Poverty: the rich continue to get richer*. Columbus, OH, and Greenbelt, MD, American Society of Criminology (ASC) Division on Critical Criminology, and the Academy of Criminal Justice Sciences (ACJS) Section on Critical Criminal Justice (http://critcrim.org/summarizing_the_new_us_census_bureau_report_on_income_and_poverty_the_rich_continue_to_get_richer, accessed 18 July 2009).

23. WHO and UNICEF Joint Monitoring Programme for Water Supply and Sanitation. *Progress on drinking water and sanitation*. New York, NY, and Geneva, UNICEF and the World Health Organization, 2008.

24. *The situation of women and girls: facts and figures*. New York, NY, United Nations Children's Fund, 2009.

25. Campbell JC. Health consequences of intimate partner violence. *Lancet*, 2002, 359:1331–1336. PMID:11965295 doi:10.1016/S0140-6736(02)08336-8

26. Plichta SB, Falik M. Prevalence of violence and its implications for women's health. *Women's Health Issues*, 2001, 11:244–258. PMID:11336864 doi:10.1016/S1049-3867(01)00085-8

27. *Gender and health in disasters*. Geneva, World Health Organization, 2002 (http://www.who.int/gender/other_health/en/genderdisasters.pdf, accessed 18 July 2009).

28. *Mainstreaming gender into disaster recovery and reconstruction*. Washington, DC, The World Bank, 2007 (http://www.preventionweb.net/files/8024_MainstreamingGenderintoDisasterRecoveryandRecostruct.txt, accessed 18 July 2009).

29. Cottingham J, Garcia-Moreno C, Reis C. Sexual and reproductive health in conflict areas: the imperative to address violence against women. *BJOG: An International Journal of Obstetrics and Gynaecology*, 2008, 115:301–303. PMID:18190365 doi:10.1111/j.1471-0528.2007.01605.x

30. Garcia-Moreno C, Reis C. Overview on women's health in crises. *Health in emergencies* (newsletter). Issue No. 20 "Focus: Women's health". Geneva, World Health Organization, January 2005 (http://www.who.int/entity/hac/network/newsletter/Final_HiE_n20_%20Jan_2005_finalpdf.pdf, accessed 18 July 2009).

31. *The world health report 2003: shaping the future*. Geneva, World Health Organization, 2003.

32. Gupta N et al. Assessing human resources for health: what can be learned from labour force surveys? *Human Resources for Health*, 2003, 1:5 (http://www.human-resources-health.com/content/1/1/5, accessed 18 July 2009). PMID:12904250 doi:10.1186/1478-4491-1-5

33. Lavallée R, Hanvoravongchai P, Gupta N. The use of population census data for gender analysis of the health workforce. In: Dal Poz MR, Gupta N, Quain E, Soucat A, eds. *Handbook on monitoring and evaluation of human resources for health*. Geneva, World Health Organization, World Bank and United States Agency for International Development (in press).

34. George A. *Human resources for health: a gender analysis*. Paper commissioned by the Women and Gender Equity Knowledge Network. Geneva, World Health Organization, 2007 (http://www.who.int/social_determinants/resources/human_resources_for_health_wgkn_2007.pdf, accessed 18 July 2009).

35. *Gender and health workforce statistics*. Geneva, World Health Organization, 2008 (http://www.who.int/hrh/statistics/spotlight_2.pdf, accessed 18 July 2009).

36. *The world health report 2006: working together for health*. Geneva, World Health Organization, 2006.

37. Prüss-Üstün A, Rapiti E, Hutin Y. *Sharps injuries – global burden of disease from sharps injuries to health-care workers*. Geneva, World Health Organization, 2003.

38. Aiken LH et al. Hospital nurse staffing and patient mortality, nurse burnout, and job dissatisfaction. *Journal of the American Medical Association*, 2002, 288:1987–1993. PMID:12387650 doi:10.1001/jama.288.16.1987

39. Josephson M, Lagerstrom M, Hagberg M, Wigaeus EH. Musculoskeletal symptoms and job strain among nursing personnel: a study over a three year period. *Occupational and Environmental Medicine*, 1997, 54:681–685. PMID:9423583 doi:10.1136/oem.54.9.681

40. Mayhew C. Occupational violence: a neglected occupational health and safety issue? *Policy and Practice in Health and Safety*, 2003, 1:31–58.

41. Seifert A, Dagenais L. *Vivre avec les microbes: la prévention et le contrôle des infections professionnelles*. Montréal, Confédération des syndicats nationaux, 1998.

42. Pechter E et al. Work-related asthma among health care workers: Surveillance data from California, Massachusetts, Michigan, and New Jersey, 1993–1997. *American Journal of Industrial Medicine*, 2005, 47:265–275. PMID:15712261 doi:10.1002/ajim.20138

CHAPTER 2

THE GIRL CHILD

The world has 1.2 billion children under the age of 10 years, and more than 50% of them live in Asia. Children today live in smaller families than they did 30 or 40 years ago because the average number of children per woman has declined significantly (see Chapter 1). The health and development of these children is a prime concern for all societies. The health and well-being of young girls is of particular concern because of their future reproductive roles and the clear intergenerational effects that poor maternal health has on the health and development prospects of their children.

Still too many deaths of infants and children

The past 50 years have seen a dramatic decline in mortality in children. Nevertheless, millions of children die prematurely, and childhood continues to be a time of vulnerability to a wide range of health risks. The burden of disease is particularly severe in Africa, but is also significant in the Eastern Mediterranean and South-East Asia regions (Figure 1). Globally, the leading causes of death and disability in girls under 10 years of age are communicable diseases (respiratory tract infections and diarrhoea) and neonatal conditions (low birth weight, birth asphyxia and trauma) which together account for over 60% of the total (Table 1).[a]

Most deaths in children under the age of 10 take place before they reach their fifth birthday. Despite considerable improvements in child survival over the past two decades, every year some nine million children under five years, including 4.3 million girls,[2] die from conditions that are largely preventable and treatable. The main causes of these deaths are prematurity and low birth weight (11%), neonatal infections (11%), diarrhoeal diseases (17%), and post-neonatal acute respiratory infections, mainly pneumonia (18%) (Figure 2). It is estimated that 200 million children under five years of age fail to reach their full potential because of poor health.[4]

Malnutrition is both a direct cause of child deaths and an underlying cause of many more (see below and Figure 2). In addition to malnutrition (undernutrition), other leading risk factors for child mortality and ill-health include unsafe water, poor sanitation and hygiene, suboptimal breastfeeding, and indoor smoke from solid fuels (Table 2). Climate change is likely to affect the basic requirements for maintaining child health, namely clean air and water,

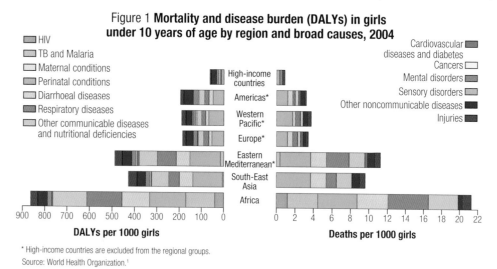

Figure 1 **Mortality and disease burden (DALYs) in girls under 10 years of age by region and broad causes, 2004**

HIV
TB and Malaria
Maternal conditions
Perinatal conditions
Diarrhoeal diseases
Respiratory diseases
Other communicable diseases and nutritional deficiencies

Cardiovascular diseases and diabetes
Cancers
Mental disorders
Sensory disorders
Other noncommunicable diseases
Injuries

High-income countries
Americas*
Western Pacific*
Europe*
Eastern Mediterranean*
South-East Asia
Africa

900 800 700 600 500 400 300 200 100 0
DALYs per 1000 girls

0 2 4 6 8 10 12 14 16 18 20 22
Deaths per 1000 girls

* High-income countries are excluded from the regional groups.
Source: World Health Organization.[1]

a Conditions arising during the perinatal period include low birth weight, birth asphyxia and birth trauma, and other perinatal conditions.

Table 1 **Ten leading causes of death in females aged 0–9 years by country income group, 2004**

	World					Low-income countries		
Rank	**Cause**	**Deaths (000s)**	**%**		**Rank**	**Cause**	**Deaths (000s)**	**%**
1	Lower respiratory infections	948	17.6		1	Lower respiratory infections	807	18.8
2	Diarrhoeal diseases	858	15.9		2	Diarrhoeal diseases	720	16.8
3	Prematurity and low birth weight	567	10.5		3	Neonatal infections*	426	9.9
4	Neonatal infections*	545	10.1		4	Prematurity and low birth weight	405	9.4
5	Birth asphyxia and birth trauma	411	7.6		5	Malaria	372	8.7
6	Malaria	397	7.4		6	Birth asphyxia and birth trauma	312	7.3
7	Measles	201	3.7		7	Measles	187	4.4
8	Congenital anomalies	188	3.5		8	Pertussis	118	2.8
9	HIV/AIDS	138	2.5		9	Congenital anomalies	115	2.7
10	Pertussis	125	2.3		10	HIV/AIDS	107	2.5

	Middle-income countries					High-income countries		
Rank	**Cause**	**Deaths (000s)**	**%**		**Rank**	**Cause**	**Deaths (000s)**	**%**
1	Prematurity and low birth weight	155	14.6		1	Congenital anomalies	9	21.7
2	Lower respiratory infections	139	13.1		2	Prematurity and low birth weight	7	17.3
3	Diarrhoeal diseases	137	12.9		3	Neonatal infections*	6	14.6
4	Neonatal infections*	113	10.7		4	Birth asphyxia and birth trauma	3	7.6
5	Birth asphyxia and birth trauma	96	9.0		5	Lower respiratory infections	2	4.2
6	Congenital anomalies	63	6.0		6	Diarrhoeal diseases	1	3.4
7	HIV/AIDS	30	2.8		7	Road traffic accidents	1	3.3
8	Malaria	25	2.3		8	Endocrine disorders	1	2.8
9	Meningitis	21	2.0		9	Violence	1	1.6
10	Drownings	19	1.8		10	Drownings	1	1.2

*Includes severe neonatal infections and other non-infectious causes arising in the perinatal period.
Source: World Health Organization.[1]

sufficient food and adequate shelter. Many of the biggest global killers are highly sensitive to climatic conditions. More than three million deaths each year are caused by a combination of malaria, diarrhoea and protein-energy malnutrition.[5]

A very large proportion of child deaths take place very early in life, usually within the first month. Deaths in this neonatal period[a] represent nearly half of child deaths in all regions apart from the African Region. As overall levels of child mortality decline, the proportion of total deaths during the neonatal period tends to increase. To a significant extent, this is because critical interventions during this period depend on a well functioning health system that is able to deliver high-quality care to pregnant women and their newborn infants, but access to such care is unattainable in many settings.[6]

Inequalities in child mortality relate primarily to income: children living in poor countries are far more likely to die prematurely than those living in wealthier countries; and within a country, children living in poor households are more likely to die than those living in richer ones.

---

a Conditions arising in the first 28 days of life (the neonatal period) include prematurity and low birth weight, birth asphyxia and birth trauma, and other perinatal conditions.

Sex differentials in health

Globally, girls are not more likely to die under the age of five years than boys are. In fact, girls may have a certain advantage (Figure 3). However, in a few countries (including China and India) mortality rates for children under five years are higher among girls than boys.[2] Data from household surveys over the past 20 years indicate that the female disadvantage has tended to persist in India and may have worsened in some other countries such as Nepal and Pakistan. By contrast, recently released data for Bangladesh show that the gap has narrowed significantly over time and females under five years currently have lower mortality rates than males.[7]

Although there are some differences between girls and boys in terms of access to key elements of care during childhood, these are generally not systematic or uniform within regions or countries, either across interventions or across countries and regions. For instance, available data on immunization coverage show that while significant sex differentials in coverage in different countries do occur, there is no overall systematic bias against either boys or girls (Figure 3). In some countries immunization coverage is higher for boys, while in others it is higher for girls. However, there is evidence that boys are more likely to suffer from severe malnutrition (stunting) than girls are.

Undernutrition is the underlying cause of 3.5 million child deaths and accounts for 35% of the disease burden in children under five years (Figure 2).[8] Malnutrition is often acute in populations affected by humanitarian crises.[9]

Lack of access to nutritious foods, especially in the present context of rising food prices, is a common direct cause of malnutrition. Poor feeding practices, such as inadequate breastfeeding and offering insufficient or less nutritious food, are major contributory factors. Indirect causes of malnutrition actually account for a higher toll of mortality and burden of disease than the direct causes.[10] An important indirect cause is infection – particularly frequent or persistent diarrhoea, pneumonia, measles and malaria – which undermines a child's nutritional status.[11] In particular, severe diarrhoea leads to fluid loss and may

Table 2 **Leading risk factors for mortality in girls under five years of age, 2004**

Risk	Low-income countries	Middle-income countries	High-income countries
	Deaths per 100 000 children		
Childhood underweight	641	71	2
Unsafe water, sanitation, hygiene	410	98	4
Suboptimal breastfeeding	302	111	17
Indoor smoke from solid fuels	248	32	0
Vitamin A deficiency	180	31	1
Zinc deficiency	119	21	1

Source: World Health Organization.[3]

Figure 2 **Distribution of major causes of death in girls under five years of age, including disease-specific contribution of undernutrition, 2004**

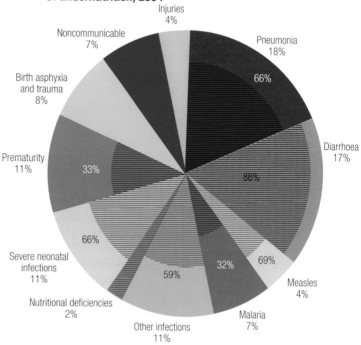

Shaded area indicates contribution of undernutrition to each cause of death.
Source: World Health Organization.[3]

Figure 3 **Sex differences in key child health indicators, selected countries, 2002–2007**

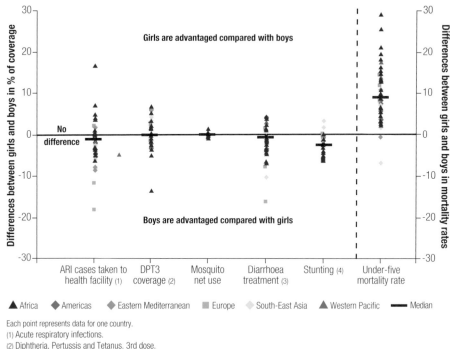

Each point represents data for one country.
(1) Acute respiratory infections.
(2) Diphtheria, Pertussis and Tetanus. 3rd dose.
(3) Oral rehydration salts (ORS) or recommended homemade solutions (RHS).
(4) Height-for-age less than minus two standard deviations from the median of the reference population.

Source: Demographic and Health Surveys in 43 countries (data was available in 31 countries for stunting and in 14 countries for mosquito net use), 2002–2007.

be life-threatening, especially in young children and people who are malnourished or have impaired immunity. Underweight children are also more vulnerable to almost all infectious diseases and have a lower prognosis for full recovery.

Risk factors for such infections include unsafe water, inadequate sanitation and insufficient hygiene. It has been estimated that 88% of cases of diarrhoea worldwide are attributable to unsafe water, inadequate sanitation or insufficient hygiene.[10] An estimated 860 000 deaths per year in children under five years of age are caused directly and indirectly by malnutrition that is induced by unsafe water, inadequate sanitation and insufficient hygiene.[10]

Malnutrition among pregnant women can lead to premature and low-birth-weight babies, putting them at risk of poor health and early and premature death, and of learning disabilities later in life.[12,13]

Undernutrition is one aspect of malnutrition. At the same time, increasing rates of overweight and obesity among children worldwide represent major risks for poor health in adulthood. In some countries, up to 20% of children under the age of five years are overweight (e.g. Albania, Lesotho, Ukraine)[14] and in a few countries (Albania, Bosnia and Herzegovina, Ukraine) more than 10% of children under five years are obese. In both developed and developing countries, girls under five years and adolescent girls are more likely to be overweight than boys (see also next chapter).[15–17]

Female genital mutilation

Girls and women face particular health risks due to harmful practices such as female genital mutilation (FGM). Millions of girls and women are estimated to have undergone FGM, which involves partial or total removal of the female external genitalia or other injury to the female genital organs for nonmedical reasons.[18]

It is estimated that 92.5 million girls and women above the age of 10 years in Africa are living with the consequences of FGM. Of these, 12.5 million are girls between 10 and 14 years of age.[19] Each year, some three million girls in Africa are subjected to FGM.[20] Although available data are incomplete, it appears that there have been small decreases in the extent of FGM in recent years. However, the data indicate a growing tendency for FGM to be carried out by health professionals, a decline in the average age at which FGM is performed, and a marked increase in the proportion of girls who undergo FGM before the age of five years.

Abuse and maltreatment

Many children of both sexes suffer from physical and emotional maltreatment, sexual abuse, neglect and negligent treatment, and commercial or other exploitation. Although reliable and comprehensive data are limited, the evidence that is available indicates that girls are far more likely than boys to suffer sexual abuse. A review of evidence generated estimates of prevalence of different types of sexual abuse in children and young people up to the age of 18 years as follows:

- non-contact sexual abuse (3.1% boys, 6.8% girls);
- contact sexual abuse (3.7% boys, 13.2% girls);
- penetrative sexual abuse (1.9% boys, 5.3% girls);
- any sexual abuse (8.7% boys, 25.3% girls).[21]

Child abuse has both immediate and long-term consequences for the health of women and contributes significantly to depression, alcohol and drug use and dependence, panic disorder, post-traumatic stress disorder, and suicide attempts.[21] In emergency and refugee settings, girls may be at particular risk of sexual violence, exploitation and abuse by combatants, security forces, members of their communities, aid workers and others.[22]

Conclusion

The health of the adults of tomorrow is critically dependent on the health of the children of today. While the girl child benefits from a number of biological advantages in terms of her survival and health, she also faces social, cultural and gender-based disadvantages that place her health at risk. Many of the health problems faced by adult women have their origins in childhood. These include poor nutrition, which is particularly important because of its intergenerational repercussions. Preventing child abuse and neglect and ensuring a supportive environment in early childhood will help girls to achieve optimal physical, social and emotional development and will avoid a significant burden of disease associated with chronic diseases, including mental health disorders and substance use, later in life.

Summary findings and implications

■ Considerable advances have been made in child health, and girls have a much greater chance of surviving childhood than they had several decades ago. However, progress has been uneven, especially in the poorest countries. Progress has been slowest in countries affected by high levels of HIV/AIDS and conflict. Pneumonia and diarrhoea – conditions that are readily preventable and treatable – continue to kill more than three million girls under the age of five every year.

■ Malnutrition is an important determinant of health, both in childhood and beyond. The nutritional status of girls is of particular importance due to their future reproductive role and the intergenerational effects of poor female nutrition.

■ Girls and women may face particular health risks due to harmful practices. Over 100 million girls and women have been subjected to FGM. The evidence indicates that, despite some declines in overall prevalence, the procedure is being increasingly medicalized and carried out at younger ages.

■ Girls are far more likely than boys to have been subjected to sexual abuse, with one girl in four reporting such abuse in the course of their lives.

■ To address these problems, attention must be directed to priority interventions, including safe childbirth, improvement of nutritional status, access to immunization and health care for childhood diseases, integrated approaches to address child abuse and maltreatment, and ensuring a supportive early childhood environment that will help girls to achieve optimal physical, social and emotional development. Political, legal and social interventions are also needed to eliminate FGM and other harmful practices. There must be attention to the physical and psychosocial needs of children growing up amid humanitarian crises.

References

1. *The global burden of disease: 2004 update.* Geneva, World Health Organization, 2008.
2. *World health statistics 2009.* Geneva, World Health Organization, 2009.
3. *Global health risks: mortality and burden of disease attributable to selected major risks.* Geneva, World Health Organization (in press).
4. Grantham-McGregor S et al., International Child Development Steering Group. Developmental potential in the first 5 years for children in developing countries. *Lancet*, 2007, 369:60–70. PMID:17208643 doi:10.1016/S0140-6736(07)60032-4
5. *Protecting health from climate change* (World Health Day campaign for 2008). Geneva, World Health Organization, 2008 (http://www.who.int/world-health-day/previous/2008/en/index.html, accessed 18 July 2009).
6. *The world health report 2005: make every mother and child count.* Geneva, World Health Organization, 2005 (http://www.who.int/whr/2005/chapter5/en/, accessed 18 July 2009).
7. STATcompiler. *Demographic and Health Surveys in four countries between 1990 and 2007.* Calverton, MD, ICF Macro (http://www.statcompiler.com).
8. Black RE et al. Maternal and child undernutrition: global and regional exposures and health consequences. *Lancet*, 2008, 371:243–260. PMID:18207566 doi:10.1016/S0140-6736(07)61690-0
9. *Women, girls, boys & men – different needs, equal opportunities. Gender handbook for humanitarian action.* Geneva, Inter-agency Standing Committee, 2006 (http://www. humanitarianreform.org/Default.aspx?tabid=659, accessed 8 June 2009).

10. Prüss-Ustün A, Bos R, Gore F, Bartram J. *Safe water, better health – costs, benefits and sustainability of interventions to protect and promote health.* Geneva, World Health Organization, 2008. (http://whqlibdoc.who.int/publications/2008/9789241596435_eng.pdf, accessed 18 July 2009).

11. Child and adolescent health and development – malnutrition. Geneva, World Health Organization, 2009 (http://www.who.int/child_adolescent_health/topics/prevention_care/child/nutrition/malnutrition/en/index.html, accessed 8 June 2009).

12. Berkman DS et al. Effects of stunting, diarrhoeal disease, and parasitic infection during infancy on cognition in late childhood: a follow-up study. *Lancet*, 2002, 359:564–571. PMID:11867110 doi:10.1016/S0140-6736(02)07744-9

13. Mendez MA, Adair LS. Serverity and timing of stunting in the first two years of life affect performance on cognitive tests in late childhood. *The Journal of Nutrition*, 1999, 129:1555–1562. PMID:10419990

14. WHO global database on child growth and malnutrition, Geneva, 2009 (http://www.who.int/nutgrowthdb).

15. Kelishadi R et al. Obesity and associated modifiable environmental factors in Iranian adolescents: Isfahan Healthy Heart Program - Heart Health Promotion from Childhood. *Pediatrics International*, 2003, 45:435–442. PMID:12911481 doi:10.1046/j.1442-200X.2003.01738.x

16. al-Nuaim AR, Bamgboye EA, al-Herbish A. The pattern of growth and obesity in Saudi Arabian male school children. *International Journal of Obesity and Related Metabolic Disorders*, 1996, 20:1000–1005. PMID:8923156

17. McCarthy HD, Ellis SM, Cole TJ. Central overweight and obesity in British youth aged 11-16 years: cross sectional surveys of waist circumference. *BMJ (Clinical Research Ed.)*, 2003, 326:624. PMID:12649234 doi:10.1136/bmj.326.7390.624

18. *Eliminating female genital mutilation: an interagency statement.* Geneva, World Health Organization, 2008 (http://web.unfpa.org/upload/lib_pub_file/756_filename_fgm.pdf, accessed 18 July 2009).

19. Yoder PS, Khan S. *Numbers of women circumcised in Africa: the production of a total.* Calverton, MD, Macro International Inc., 2007.

20. *Changing a harmful social convention: female genital mutilation/cutting.* Innocenti Digest, No. 12. Florence, UNICEF, 2005.

21. Andrews G et al. Child sexual abuse. In: Ezzati M, Lopez A, Rodgers A, Murray C, eds. *Comparative quantification of health risks: global and regional burden of disease attributable to selected major risk factors.* Vol. 2. Geneva, World Health Organization, 2004.

22. Garcia Moreno C, Reis C. Overview on women's health in crises. *Health in emergencies* (newsletter). Issue No. 20 "Focus: Women's health". Geneva, World Health Organization, January 2005 (http://www.who.int/entity/hac/network/newsletter/Final_HiE_n20_%20Jan_2005_finalpdf.pdf).

CHAPTER

3

ADOLESCENT GIRLS

Adolescence is usually a time of good health for girls, with opportunities for growth and development. But it can also be a time of risk, particularly with regard to sexual activity and substance use. Preventing and dealing with such risks is essential for the health of young people now and for their health in future years.

Worldwide there are some 1.2 billion adolescents aged between 10 and 19 years. Around 90% of them live in developing countries, and approximately 600 million are female.[1] The health and development of these girls is very important now, and continues to be important as they mature into adults. The health of adolescents sets the stage for their future health and well-being, as well as for the health of their children and the development of their societies.

A time of good health but also risk

Adolescence is normally characterized by low levels of disease and death; it is the period of life when mortality rates are lowest. However, it is also a time of huge physical, social and emotional changes. In many settings, girls are not given the support they need to deal with these changes. The societies in which they live are unable to provide optimal conditions for their healthy development. As a result, girls may miss opportunities to progress successfully through the transition to adulthood, becoming vulnerable to behaviours that put their health at risk.

The highest rates of mortality and burden of disease in adolescent girls are found in Africa and South-East Asia (Figure 1). Deaths from suicide and injuries associated with road traffic accidents and burns figure prominently as causes of death around the world.[2] Communicable diseases including HIV/AIDS are important causes of death, especially in Africa. In all regions, adolescent girls face significant burdens of disease associated with mental health problems.[2] In high-income countries in the Americas, Europe and Western Pacific regions, neuropsychiatric conditions, such as unipolar depressive disorders, schizophrenia and bipolar disorders,[2] are responsible for a large share of the burden of ill-health among female adolescents In the Eastern Mediterranean and South-East Asia regions, injuries stand alongside neuropsychiatric problems in terms of their impact on disease burden. In high- and middle-income countries in general, road traffic accidents are the leading cause of death among adolescent

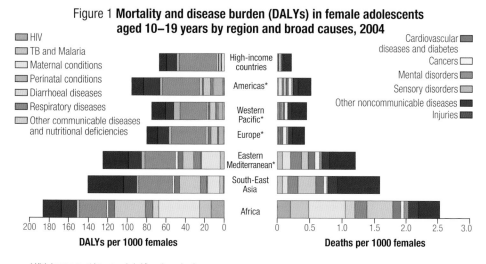

Figure 1 **Mortality and disease burden (DALYs) in female adolescents aged 10–19 years by region and broad causes, 2004**

* High-income countries are excluded from the regional groups.
Source: World Health Organization.[2]

females, whereas respiratory tract infections and other communicable diseases dominate in low-income countries (Table 1).

Puberty and sexual debut

For girls, the onset of puberty is the most obvious signal of the start of their sexual and reproductive lives. Girls' experiences during this period, and the opportunities and protection that their cultures and societies provide, can make the difference in their lives between good health and the ability to contribute fully to society on the one hand, and suboptimal functioning marked by harmful behaviours that lead to ill-health and unhappiness on the other.

Many adolescent girls face constraints and marginalization as a result of poverty, harmful social and cultural traditions, humanitarian crises and geographical isolation. These factors hinder their access to information, education, health care and economic opportunities.[3] At precisely the time when they are most in need of support that could help protect them from health risks, in some settings adolescent girls are pressured into early marriage and childbearing. A full 38% of girls in developing countries, notably in Asia, marry before the age of 18, and 14% before the age of 15.[3]

Table 1 **Ten leading causes of death in females aged 10–19 years by country income group, 2004**

World				Low-income countries			
Rank	Cause	Deaths (000s)	%	Rank	Cause	Deaths (000s)	%
1	Lower respiratory infections	57	8.9	1	Lower respiratory infections	49	10.6
2	Road traffic accidents	37	5.6	2	Self-inflicted injuries	24	5.2
3	Self-inflicted injuries	36	5.5	3	Fires	21	4.6
4	Tuberculosis	29	4.5	4	Tuberculosis	21	4.5
5	Fires	24	3.8	5	Meningitis	18	3.9
6	Drownings	23	3.5	6	HIV/AIDS	17	3.7
7	Meningitis	21	3.3	7	Malaria	16	3.4
8	HIV/AIDS	20	3.0	8	Road traffic accidents	16	3.4
9	Malaria	17	2.7	9	Diarrhoeal diseases	12	2.6
10	Diarrhoeal diseases	14	2.2	10	Drownings	11	2.4

Middle-income countries				High-income countries			
Rank	Cause	Deaths (000s)	%	Rank	Cause	Deaths (000s)	%
1	Road traffic accidents	17	9.9	1	Road traffic accidents	4	28.9
2	Drownings	11	6.8	2	Self-inflicted injuries	1	9.5
3	Self-inflicted injuries	10	6.2	3	Violence	1	5.0
4	Tuberculosis	8	4.7	4	Leukaemia	1	4.2
5	Lower respiratory infections	8	4.5	5	Congenital anomalies	1	4.2
6	Leukaemia	6	3.8	6	Endocrine disorders	0	3.1
7	Violence	5	3.0	7	Poisonings	0	2.0
8	Congenital anomalies	4	2.6	8	Lower respiratory infections	0	1.5
9	Poisonings	4	2.4	9	Stroke	0	1.5
10	Fires	3	1.8	10	Epilepsy	0	1.3

Source: World Health Organization.[2]

Contrary to popular belief, there is little evidence at the global level that girls today have their first sexual encounters at younger ages than in the past. Almost everywhere in the world, girls' first sexual activity occurs during late adolescence – between the ages of 15 and 19 years.[4] Unfortunately, for many girls early sexual activity is associated with coercion or even violence.[5] The younger the woman is at first sex, the greater the likelihood that her sexual initiation is forced.[5] Female adolescents are exposed to unwanted pregnancy and to sexually transmitted infections, including HIV, and they experience long-term mental and physical health consequences.

Few young women use a contraceptive of any kind at their first sexual experience.[6] Their access to contraception is limited by their own lack of information and skills, and by the fact that most reproductive health-care services in developing countries are designed to serve the needs of married women of reproductive age.[7]

Adolescent pregnancy

Adolescent birth rates have been declining globally but they remain high in parts of Africa and Asia.[8] Adolescent pregnancy is more common in adolescents who live in poverty and in rural areas, and it is more likely to occur among the less educated (Figure 2).

For several reasons pregnancy and childbirth are more risky for very young adolescents. In developing countries, complications of pregnancy and childbirth are the leading cause of death in young women aged between 15 and 19 years. About 15% of total maternal deaths worldwide, and 26% in Africa, occur among adolescents.[9] The adverse health effects of adolescent childbearing are reflected in the poor health of their infants: perinatal deaths are 50% higher among babies born to mothers under 20 years of age than among those born to mothers aged 20–29 years. Moreover, babies of adolescent mothers are more likely to have low birth weight, which is a risk factor for ill-health during infancy.[10]

Because many adolescents face unwanted pregnancy, rates of unsafe abortion among young women are high, especially in Africa where girls aged 15–19 years account for one in every four unsafe abortions.[11] Even when they do not result in death, the immediate and long-term health consequences of such interventions – which include haemorrhage, reproductive tract infections and infertility – can be severe.

Sexually transmitted infections

Young women are particularly vulnerable to HIV infection, due to a combination of biological factors, lack of access to information and services, and social norms and values that undermine their ability to protect themselves. Their vulnerability may increase during humanitarian crises and emergencies when economic hardship can lead to increased risk of exploitation, such as trafficking, and increased reproductive health risks related to the exchange of sex for money and other necessities.

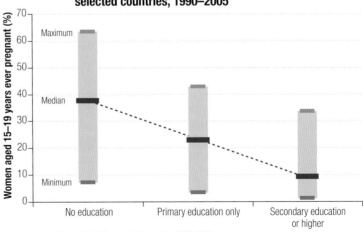

Figure 2 **Adolescence pregnancy rates by educational level, selected countries, 1990–2005**

Source: Demographic and Health Surveys in 55 countries, 1990–2005.

Figure 3 **HIV prevalence among adolescents aged 15–19 years, by sex, selected countries in sub-Saharan Africa, 2001–2007**

Adolescents aged 15–19 years living with HIV (%)

■ Male ■ Female

Senegal 2005, Ghana 2003, Mali 2006, Rwanda 2005, Ethiopia 2005, Burkina Faso 2003, Guinea 2005, Liberia 2007, United Republic of Tanzania 2007–08, Cameroon 2004, Uganda 2004–05, Kenya 2003, Zambia 2007–08, Zimbabwe 2005–06, Lesotho 2004, Swaziland 2006–07

Source: Demographic and Health Surveys in 16 countries, sub-Saharan Africa, 2001–2007.

Young women tend to have sex with older men who are more sexually experienced and more likely to be infected with HIV. In most African countries that have data, adolescent girls are much more likely to be infected than young men of the same age (see Chapter 4) (Figure 3). Although many young girls have heard about HIV/AIDS, only 38% are able to describe correctly the main ways to avoid infection. Only a minority use condoms when having high-risk sex and fewer still are aware of their HIV status.[7,12] This is perhaps not surprising since programmes for HIV prevention, information and services directed at young people have generally been poorly implemented.[12]

Substance use

Unsafe sexual activity is by no means the only important risk factor in adolescent girls. In several European countries, alcohol consumption increased among female adolescents between 1993 and 2003.[13] Meanwhile, data from 37 low- and middle-income countries indicate that 14% of girls aged 13–15 years reported drinking alcohol in the past month compared to 18% of boys.[14] Because of male–female differences in body weight and body water content, girls are more vulnerable than boys to the psychoactive effects of alcohol and are therefore more likely to suffer the consequences of its use – including violence, unintentional injuries and vulnerability to sexual coercion.[15]

Like adolescent boys, many girls take up smoking during adolescence and there is evidence that tobacco advertising is increasingly targeting girls and women.[16] Data from 151 countries indicate that approximately 10% of adolescents (12% among boys and 7% among girls) smoke cigarettes and 10% use tobacco products other than cigarettes (e.g. pipes, water pipes, smokeless tobacco, and *bidis*).[17] Smoking among girls is more common in high-income countries than in lower income countries.[18]

Poor diet and physical inactivity

Poor diet and physical inactivity are major risk factors for chronic diseases, leading to premature death and disability in adulthood. Adolescence is a time when girls start to take decisions about the food they eat and the physical activity they engage in (although in impoverished communities their choices are limited). Poor habits can lead to overweight and obesity. Obese adolescents tend to grow up to be obese adults and are thus exposed to a higher risk of diseases, such as osteoarthritis, diabetes and cardiovascular diseases, at a younger age than those who are not obese.[19] While adolescent girls in many countries still suffer from undernutrition, data from 20 low- and middle-income countries show that around 12% of school-going 13–15-year-old girls are overweight.[20]

Physical activity is not only crucial to avoiding weight gain but is also an important factor in improving adolescents' control over anxiety and depression. Physically active adolescents more readily adopt other healthy behaviours – including avoiding tobacco, alcohol and drug use – and show higher academic performance at school.[20] However, data from 36 low- and middle-income countries indicate that 86% of girls do not meet recommended levels of physical activity, which is a far higher proportion than among boys (Figure 4).

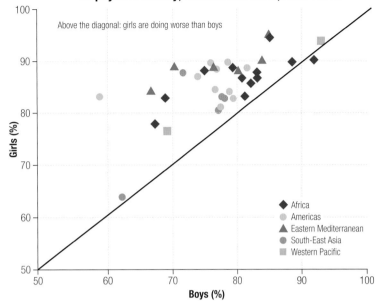

Figure 4 **Students aged 13–15 not meeting recommended levels of physical activity, selected countries, 2003–2008**

Each point represents data for one country.
Source: Global School-based Student Health Surveys in 36 countries, 2003–2008.

Mental health in adolescence

Since adolescence is a time of social, emotional and physical change, it is perhaps not surprising to find that young women are at significant risk of mental health problems such as unipolar depressive disorders, schizophrenia and bipolar disorders.[2] The risk factors driving these disorders go well beyond adolescent identity crises or peer pressure; they include exposure to violence (childhood sexual abuse, parental domestic violence, corporal punishment at school, bullying and sexual coercion), the devaluation or restriction of girls' opportunities, and poverty (especially where this affects the adolescent's ability to attend school).[21] Lack of care for such conditions during adolescence can have serious repercussions as young people grow into adulthood and older age. This issue is also dealt with in Chapters 5 and 6.

Conclusion

Adolescence is a crucial time for girls today and profoundly influences the women and mothers that they will become tomorrow. The behaviours developed during adolescence are often determined by the social and economic environment in which adolescents grow up. Today, these environments are too often neither safe nor supportive. Actions are needed to ensure that societies and their health systems respond appropriately to the health and development needs of adolescent girls.

Summary findings and implications

■ For girls, adolescence is generally a time of good health and of opportunities for growth and development. However, injuries, road traffic accidents, and HIV/AIDS contribute significantly to deaths and disabilities in this age group. Maternal mortality is the leading cause of death and disability among 15–19-year-old young women in developing countries.

■ During adolescence, mental health problems contribute significantly to morbidity and mortality and, if unrecognized, may render adolescents vulnerable to poor psychological and social functioning in the immediate and longer term.

■ Adolescent girls are at risk of unsafe and often unwanted sexual activity that leads to HIV/AIDS, sexually transmitted infections and unwanted pregnancy. Adolescent birth rates remain high in parts of Africa and Asia and pregnancy is more likely to occur among girls living in poverty and in rural areas and among the least educated. Early pregnancy and childbearing may be associated with significant health problems, including unsafe abortion. The health impact affects not only adolescents themselves but also their infants.

■ HIV infection is high in girls under 20 years of age in virtually all countries that have generalized HIV epidemics. This reflects the fact that girls generally have sexual relations with older men who are more sexually experienced and are therefore more likely to be infected themselves.

■ Adolescent girls are increasingly using tobacco and alcohol. These behaviours risk compromising their health in later life, as do poor diet and physical inactivity.

■ The implications of these findings are that it is important to ensure that adolescent girls have access to both primary and secondary education, including comprehensive skills-based sex education, and opportunities for adequate diet and physical activity. They need protection from early marriage, exploitation and abuse, including the prevention of intimate partner violence and sexual violence. Furthermore, female adolescents need to be able to access and use health services, particularly for sexual, reproductive and mental health care. Policy measures to limit tobacco and alcohol use and to improve road safety are important. Improved age and sex disaggregation of health information and intervention research will help to highlight the particular needs of adolescent girls and the approaches to address them. Societies as a whole must provide the support that girls need to deal successfully with the physical and emotional changes of adolescence and to make a healthy transition to adulthood.

References

1. *World population prospects: the 2008 revision*. New York, NY, United Nations Population Division, 2008 (http://www.un.org/esa/population/, accessed 19 March 2009).
2. *The global burden of disease: 2004 update*. Geneva, World Health Organization, 2008.
3. Levine R et al. *Girls count. A global investment and action agenda*. Washington, DC, Centre for Global Development, 2008.
4. Wellings K et al. Sexual behaviour in context: a global perspective. Lancet, 2006, 368:1706–1728. PMID:17098090 doi:10.1016/S0140-6736(06)69479-8
5. Garcia-Moreno C et al. *WHO multi-country study on women's health and domestic violence. Initial results on prevalence, health outcomes and women's responses*. Geneva: World Health Organization, 2005.
6. Lloyd CB, editor. *Growing up global. The changing transitions to adulthood*. Washington, DC, National Academies Press, 2005.
7. Khan S, Mishra V. *Youth reproductive and sexual health*. DHS comparative reports, No. 19. Calverton, MD, Macro International Inc., 2008.
8. *World fertility patterns 2008*. New York, NY, United Nations Population Division, 2009.
9. Patton GC et al. Global patterns of mortality in young people. *Lancet*. In press.
10. *Why is giving special attention to adolescents important for achieving Millennium Development Goal 5?* Adolescent pregnancy fact sheet. Geneva, World Health Organization, 2008.
11. *Unsafe abortion: global and regional estimates of the incidence of unsafe abortion and associated mortality in 2003*. 5th edition. Geneva, World Health Organization, 2007.
12. *2008 Report on the global AIDS epidemic*. Geneva, Joint United Nations Programme on HIV/ AIDS (UNAIDS), 2008.
13. *Alcohol and other drug use among students in 35 European countries*. Report of the European School Survey Project on Alcohol and Other Drugs Report 2003. Stockholm, Swedish Council for Information on Alcohol and Other Drugs, 2004.
14. *Global school-based student health survey*. Geneva, World Health Organization (http://www.who. int/chp/gshs/en/, accessed 18 June 2009).
15. *Global status report: alcohol and young people*. Geneva, World Health Organization, 2001.
16. *Sifting the evidence: gender and tobacco control*. Geneva, World Health Organization, 2007.
17. Warren CW et al. Global Youth Tobacco Surveillance, 2000–2007. MMWR. Surveillance Summaries, 2008, 57:1–28. PMID:18219269
18. *World health survey*. Geneva, World Health Organization (http://www.who.int/healthinfo/ survey/en/, accessed 18 June 2009).
19. *Why does childhood overweight and obesity matter?* Geneva, World Health Organization (http:// www.who.int/dietphysicalactivity/childhood_consequences/en/index.html, accessed 18 June 2009).
20. *Physical activity*. Geneva, World Health Organization (http://www.who.int/dietphysicalactivity/ pa/en/index.html, accessed 18 June 2009).
21. *Adolescent mental health in resource constrained settings: the evidence*. Geneva, World Health Organization (in press).

CHAPTER 4

ADULT WOMEN: THE REPRODUCTIVE YEARS

In many societies the passage of women from adolescence to adulthood has traditionally been symbolized, and to a certain degree defined, by marriage and childbearing. But as Chapter 3 showed, women are generally marrying later, having their first baby later, and living longer. Women's reproductive or fertile years are potentially rich and rewarding, and have an enormous impact on women's general health and well-being. This chapter looks at key issues in the sexual and reproductive health of women from puberty to the menopause. For statistical purposes, that period is defined here as extending from 15 to 44 years.[a]

Women's health during the reproductive years

For many women, the years between puberty and menopause offer multiple opportunities for personal fulfilment and development. However, this can also be a time of health risks specifically associated with sex and reproduction that may result in a significant burden of mortality and disability. The burden of ill-health in this age group is particularly high in Africa due to high rates of mortality and disability associated with HIV/AIDS and maternal conditions (Figure 1).

Moreover, while it takes two to make a baby, women alone face the health problems that are associated with pregnancy and childbearing and which cause 14% of deaths globally in this age group. Women also take on most of the responsibility for contraception.

Patterns of mortality during the reproductive years differ greatly between low- and high-income countries. In the latter, the three leading causes of female deaths are road traffic accidents, suicide and self-inflicted injuries, and breast cancer. Together these account for more than one in every four deaths. In contrast, the three leading causes of death in low-income countries are HIV/AIDS, maternal conditions and tuberculosis, which together account for one in every two deaths (Table 1).

Globally, the single leading risk factor for death and disability in women of reproductive age in low- and middle-income countries is unsafe sex, which can lead to sexually transmitted infections, including HIV (Table 2). Women who do not know how to protect themselves from such infections, or who are unable to do so, face increased risks of death or illness. So do those who cannot protect themselves from unwanted pregnancy or control their fertility because of lack of access to contraception. There is emerging evidence that violence against women is an important risk factor for their health, although the full dimensions of the problem remain insufficiently measured.

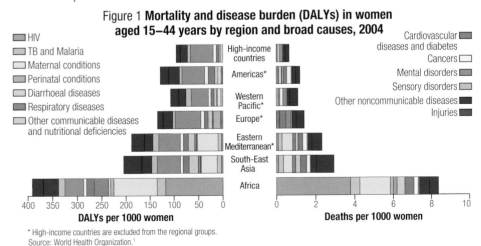

Figure 1 **Mortality and disease burden (DALYs) in women aged 15–44 years by region and broad causes, 2004**

* High-income countries are excluded from the regional groups.
Source: World Health Organization.[1]

a Some data sources use the age ranges 15–49 years or 12–44/49 years.

Pregnancy and childbearing are particularly risky for women who suffer from malnutrition – and especially anaemia. Other risk factors of growing importance include high blood pressure, high cholesterol levels, tobacco use, obesity and violence. These factors contribute to poor reproductive outcomes for both mother and infant and are direct causes of other health problems for women (see Chapter 5).

Maternal health

Throughout human history, pregnancy and childbearing have been major contributors to death and disability among women. Maternal mortality (i.e. the death of a woman during pregnancy, delivery or the postpartum period) is a key indicator of women's health and status, and shows most poignantly the difference between rich and poor, both between countries and within them. More than half a million maternal deaths occur every year and, of these, 99% happen in developing countries (Figure 2). However, there is nothing inevitable about these deaths. With the appropriate care, maternal mortality is in fact a very rare event. In industrialized countries, there are on average nine maternal deaths per 100 000 live births, whereas this figure can be as high as 1000 or more per 100 000 live births in the most disadvantaged countries. In settings where high fertility is the norm, women face such risks with each pregnancy. Thus, a woman

Table 1 Ten leading causes of death in women aged 15–44 years by country income group, 2004

World					Low-income countries			
Rank	Cause	Deaths (000s)	%		Rank	Cause	Deaths (000s)	%
1	HIV/AIDS	682	19.2		1	HIV/AIDS	494	22.3
2	Maternal conditions	516	14.6		2	Maternal conditions	434	19.5
3	Tuberculosis	228	6.4		3	Tuberculosis	161	7.3
4	Self-inflicted injuries	168	4.7		4	Lower respiratory infections	94	4.3
5	Road traffic accidents	132	3.7		5	Fires	89	4.0
6	Lower respiratory infections	121	3.4		6	Self-inflicted injuries	80	3.6
7	Ischaemic heart disease	104	2.9		7	Ischaemic heart disease	64	2.9
8	Fires	101	2.9		8	Road traffic accidents	40	1.8
9	Stroke	77	2.2		9	Stroke	32	1.5
10	Violence	61	1.7		10	Diarrhoeal diseases	30	1.3

Middle-income countries					High-income countries			
Rank	Cause	Deaths (000s)	%		Rank	Cause	Deaths (000s)	%
1	HIV/AIDS	183	15.4		1	Road traffic accidents	14	10.2
2	Maternal conditions	81	6.8		2	Self-inflicted injuries	13	9.8
3	Road traffic accidents	78	6.6		3	Breast cancer	11	7.9
4	Self-inflicted injuries	75	6.3		4	Poisonings	5	3.8
5	Tuberculosis	66	5.6		5	Stroke	5	3.6
6	Stroke	40	3.4		6	Ischaemic heart disease	4	3.2
7	Ischaemic heart disease	36	3.0		7	Violence	4	2.9
8	Breast cancer	31	2.6		8	HIV/AIDS	3	2.6
9	Violence	28	2.4		9	Trachea, bronchus and lung cancers	3	2.5
10	Lower respiratory infections	25	2.1		10	Cirrhosis of the liver	3	2.4

Source: World Health Organization.[1]

in Africa may face a lifetime risk of death during pregnancy and childbirth as high as one in 26, compared with only one in 7300 in developed regions.[3]

As deplorable as this situation is, efforts to address it are complicated by the lack of reliable data on the extent of the problem. The scant information that is available indicates that there have been declines in maternal mortality in some regions since the 1990s, notably in North Africa, East Asia, South-East Asia and Latin America and the Caribbean. The reasons for these declines are complex and specific to the local situation, but they share a number of common features, namely: increased use of contraception to delay and limit childbearing, better access to and use of high-quality health-care services, and broader social changes such as increased education and enhanced status for women. In contrast, there has been only limited progress in sub-Saharan Africa and South Asia where most of these maternal deaths continue to occur.

Countries affected by conflict or facing other forms of instability have the highest maternal and neonatal mortality rates.[4] Periods of conflict and instability bring women many additional problems such as violence, trauma and injury, disruption of primary health-care services, and poor access to health care. Such situations may also expose women to adverse environmental factors, and can lead to a shortage of health providers who may be killed, displaced, or injured.

Table 2 **Deaths in women aged 15–44 years attributable to six leading risk factors, 2004 (percentage)**

Risk	World	Low-income countries	Middle-income countries	High-income countries
	Percentage of deaths			
Unsafe sex	20	23	16	5
Unmet contraceptive need	5	6	2	0
Iron deficiency	4	5	2	0
Alcohol use	3	1	5	9
High blood pressure, cholesterol and glucose	2	2	3	4
Tobacco use	2	1	3	5
Overweight and obesity	1	1	2	4

Source: World Health Organization.[2]

Figure 2 **Maternal mortality ratios, 2005**

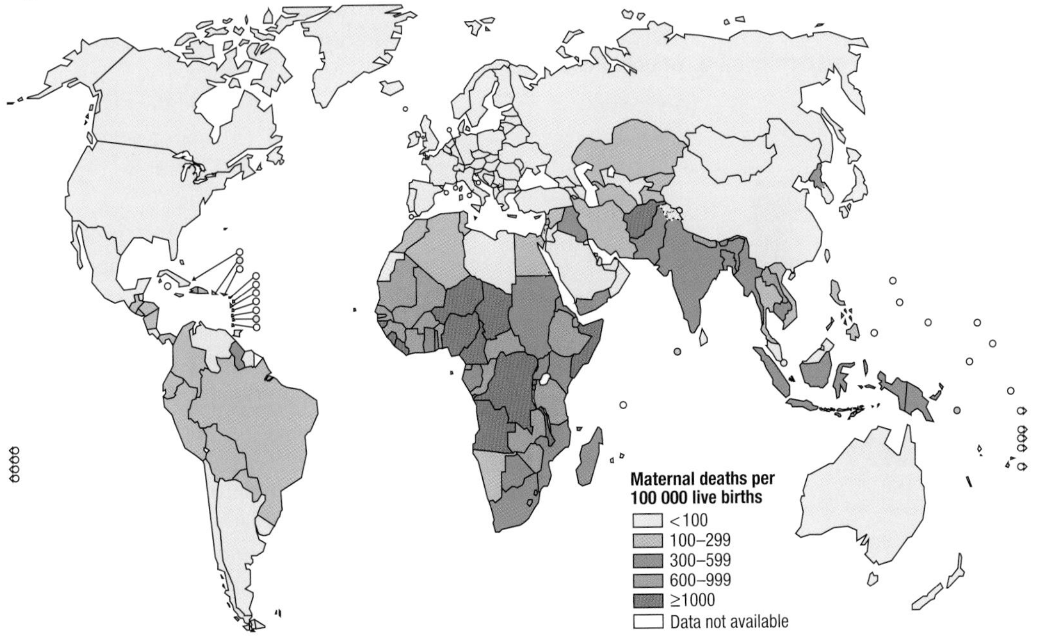

Maternal deaths per 100 000 live births
- <100
- 100–299
- 300–599
- 600–999
- ≥1000
- Data not available

Source: World Health Organization.[3]

Pregnancy and childbirth are of course not diseases. Nevertheless, they carry risks that can be reduced by health-care interventions such as the provision of family planning and maternity care and access to safe abortion care (see below). Most maternal deaths occur during or shortly after childbirth and almost all could be prevented if women were assisted at that time by a health-care professional with the necessary skills, equipment and medicines to prevent and manage complications. As noted in Chapter 1, poorer and less educated women and those living in rural areas are far less likely to give birth in the presence of a skilled health worker than better-educated women who live in wealthier households or urban areas. The reasons for this include physical inaccessibility and prohibitive costs, but may also be the result of inappropriate sociocultural practices. It is not enough for services to be available; they must also be of high quality and should be provided in a way that is both culturally appropriate and responsive to women's needs.

Despite ongoing challenges, there are some encouraging trends. Since the 1990s, in countries with trend data, the presence of skilled attendants at delivery has increased in all regions, except East and Southern Africa, with a particularly marked increase in the Middle East/North Africa.[5]

Skilled care at childbirth is but one element of the continuum of care that is required throughout and following pregnancy. Antenatal care provides opportunities for regular check-ups to assess risks, as well as to screen for and treat conditions that could affect both the woman and her baby. Delivery care ensures that obstetric emergencies are effectively managed. Postpartum care is important for detecting and treating infection and other conditions, including postpartum depression, and for providing advice on family planning. Unfortunately, at present few women receive such continuing care throughout pregnancy, childbirth and the postpartum period. Evidence from several African countries shows a dramatic drop in the coverage of care during the antenatal, delivery and postpartum periods (Figure 3).[6]

Antenatal care is particularly important because many women have nutritional deficiencies when they begin their pregnancy. Iron deficiency anaemia and deficiencies of vitamin A and iodine are commonplace. It is estimated that almost half of all pregnant women and one third of non-pregnant women worldwide have anaemia, a deficiency that significantly increases the risks to health for both mothers and infants. Maternal deficiencies in micronutrients may also affect the infant's birth weight and chance of survival, and poor vitamin A intake increases the mother's risk of night blindness.

Violence during pregnancy is common. Significant numbers of women report being physically abused during this particularly vulnerable time.[3] Violence during pregnancy is associated with an increased risk of miscarriage, stillbirth, abortion and low birth weight.[4-7]

Unsafe abortion causes a significant proportion of maternal deaths. Nearly 70 000 women die each year due to the complications of unsafe abortion. The evidence shows that women who seek an abortion will do so regardless of legal restrictions. Abortions performed in an illegal context

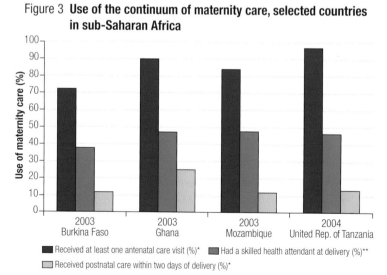

Figure 3 **Use of the continuum of maternity care, selected countries in sub-Saharan Africa**

■ Received at least one antenatal care visit (%)* ■ Had a skilled health attendant at delivery (%)**
□ Received postnatal care within two days of delivery (%)*

* Women who received ante/prenatal care for their most recent live birth.
** Deliveries in five years preceding the survey attended by skilled health personnel.

Source: Demographic and Health Surveys in selected countries, 2003–2004.

are likely to be unsafe and provided by unskilled persons in unhygienic conditions.[7] Poor women and those affected by crises and conflicts are particularly at risk. Where there are few restrictions on the availability of safe abortion, deaths and illness are dramatically reduced (Figure 4).[8]

The use of modern contraception has reduced the need for induced abortion,[7,9] yet young women, especially when they are unmarried, often face difficulty in obtaining contraception and may resort to unsafe abortion. Globally, women of all ages seek abortions but in sub-Saharan Africa, which has the highest burden of ill-health and death from unsafe abortion, one in four unsafe abortions is among adolescents aged 15–19 years.

Women's ability to plan the number and timing of the children they bear has greatly reduced the health risks associated with pregnancy and is an important success story. The use of contraception in developing countries rose from 8% in the 1960s to 62% in 2007.[10] Even so, significant unmet needs remain in all regions (Figure 5). For instance, in sub-Saharan Africa, one in four women who wish to delay or stop childbearing does not use any family planning method. Reasons for non-use include poor quality of available services, limited choice of methods, fear or experience of side-effects, and cultural or religious opposition. Gender-based barriers are also a factor, as is lack of access to services, particularly for young people, the poorer segments of the population, and those who are not married.

Women and HIV/AIDS

Globally, HIV is the leading cause of death and disease in women of reproductive age.[12] Of the 30.8 million adults living with HIV in 2007,[a] 15.5 million were women. The prevalence of HIV infection in women has increased since the early 1990s

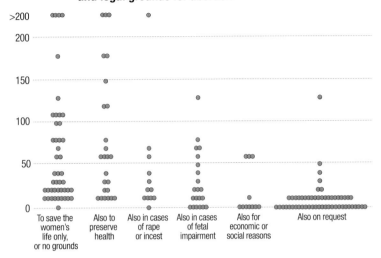

Figure 4 **Distribution of countries by numbers of deaths attributable to unsafe abortion per 100 000 live births and legal grounds for abortion**

Every dot represents one country.

Source: World Health Organization.[8]

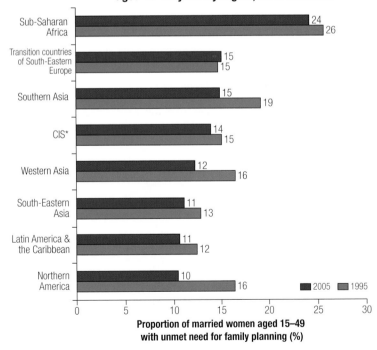

Figure 5 **Unmet need for family planning in married women aged 15–49 years by region, 1995 and 2005**

Proportion of married women aged 15–49 with unmet need for family planning (%)

* Commonwealth of Independent States (latest available data refer to a year around 2000).
Note: No data are available for Eastern Asia.
Source: United Nations.[11]

a Total number of people living with HIV/AIDS in 2007 was 33 million, including two million children younger than 15 years.

Figure 6 **HIV prevalence in women aged 15–49 years by region, 1990–2007**

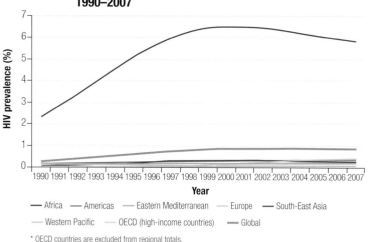

— Africa   — Americas   — Eastern Mediterranean   — Europe   — South-East Asia

— Western Pacific   — OECD (high-income countries)   — Global

* OECD countries are excluded from regional totals.

Source: UNAIDS and WHO Database 2009.

and is most marked in sub-Saharan Africa (Figure 6). Southern Africa is most affected; in 2005–2006, median HIV prevalence among pregnant women attending antenatal care was above 15% in eight Southern African countries.[a] Infection was acquired primarily through heterosexual transmission. In all regions, HIV disproportionately affects female sex workers and injecting drug users, as well as the female partners of infected males.

Women's particular vulnerability to HIV infection stems from a combination of biological factors and gender inequality. Some studies show that women are more likely than men to acquire HIV from an infected partner during unprotected heterosexual intercourse.[13] The risk posed by this biological difference is compounded in cultures that limit women's knowledge about HIV and their ability to negotiate safer sex. Stigma, violence by intimate partners, and sexual violence further increase women's vulnerability. Fewer young women than young men know that condoms can protect against HIV.[14] Furthermore, while women generally report increased condom use during high-risk sex, they are generally less likely to protect themselves than men are.[15]

The youngest women are the most vulnerable (Figure 7).[17] They not only face barriers to information about HIV – and in particular how they can protect themselves from infection – but in many settings they often engage in sexual activity with older men who are more sexually experienced and more likely to be infected.[18]

Female drug users and sex workers are particularly vulnerable; stigma, discrimination and punitive policies only increase their vulnerability.[19] The rate of HIV infection among female sex workers is high in many parts of the world, and a large proportion of women who use drugs also engage in sex work.[20] In prisons, the proportion of drug users among females is higher than among males. The use of contaminated injection equipment is particularly prevalent among women, resulting in higher rates of HIV infection.[21–24] Economic vulnerability is another key factor driving HIV infection among women. Economic vulnerability is sometimes associated with migration, which increases high-risk behaviours among women who may be driven into sex work by economic necessity.[25] On a more positive note, in recent years women have benefited from increased access to HIV prevention,

Figure 7 **HIV prevalence in women and men by age group, selected countries**

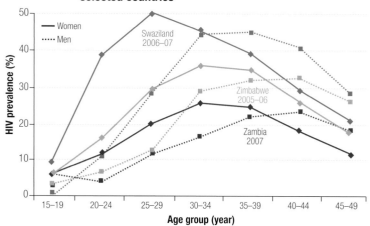

Source: Demographic and Health Surveys in selected countries, 2005–2007.[16]

a Botswana, Lesotho, Malawi, Namibia, South Africa, Swaziland, Zambia, Zimbabwe.

treatment and care.[15] Data from 90 low- and middle-income countries suggest that, overall, women are slightly advantaged in terms of access to antiretroviral therapy: at the end of 2008, 45% of women in need and only 37% of men in need received antiretroviral therapy. In 2008, 45% of pregnant women living with HIV received antiretrovirals to prevent mother-to-child transmission of HIV, up from 10% in 2004. Nonetheless, challenges remain: only 21% of pregnant women received HIV testing and counselling, and only one third of those identified as HIV-positive during antenatal care were subsequently assessed for their eligibility to receive antiretroviral therapy for their own health.

Sexually transmitted infections

The combination of biological and social factors (including humanitarian crises) that makes women more vulnerable to HIV infection also makes them far more likely than men to have sexually transmitted infections – particularly Chlamydia and trichomonas. Because the symptoms tend to be less evident in women than in men, and because women overall have more limited access to diagnosis and treatment services, women's infections are detected later and thus go longer without treatment. Delays in diagnosis and treatment, coupled with women's greater biological vulnerability to complications from untreated infection, result in women suffering far greater morbidity due to sexually transmitted infections than men do. Treatable infections – such as gonorrhoea, Chlamydia, syphilis and trichomoniasis – not only give rise to acute symptoms but also provoke chronic infection. The longer-term consequences of sexually transmitted infections include infertility, ectopic pregnancy and cancers, as well as increased vulnerability to HIV infection. Sexually transmitted infections increase the risk of adverse pregnancy outcomes, including stillbirths, low-birth-weight infants, neonatal deaths and congenital syphilis. In addition, women bear much of the stigma associated with these infections.[26]

Women in Latin America and sub-Saharan Africa are most at risk, with one in approximately four women having one of the four treatable infections at any point in time. In general, sexually transmitted infections are more common among the young, and almost half of all infected persons worldwide are aged between 15 and 24 years.[27] Women are more likely than men to be infected with genital herpes,[28] and younger women are most at risk.

Another sexually transmitted infection, the human papillomavirus (HPV), is important to women's health largely because of its relationship to cervical cancer and other genital cancers (see below). Infection with HPV is widespread and 10% of women with normal cervical cytology at any point in time are positive for HPV in the cervix. HPV is more prevalent in less developed countries where it stands at 13% overall, while in the more developed regions it is estimated to be at 8%. The highest prevalence of HPV is in Africa where it is estimated that one in five women is affected. HPV is highly transmissible, and most sexually active men and women will acquire an HPV infection at some time in their lives. Whereas most HPV infections are short-lived and benign, persistent genital infection with certain genotypes of the virus can lead to the development of ano-genital precancers, cancers and genital warts.

Cervical cancer

Cervical cancer is globally the second most common type of cancer among women and virtually all cases are linked to genital infection with HPV. There were more than 500 000 new cases of cervical cancer and 250 000 deaths from it worldwide in 2005.[1] Almost 80% of cases today occur in low-income countries, where access to cervical cancer screening and prevention services is almost non-existent (Figure 8). A highly effective vaccine against HPV is now available but cost and accessibility limit its use in less developed countries. Cervical cancer can also be prevented through regular screening coupled with treatment, but this is rarely available in most developing countries.

Infertility

Although men are just as likely to be infertile as women, their female partners are more often stigmatized and blamed when couples fail to produce offspring.[29] In high-income countries, infertility is often associated with late start of childbearing, but can be resolved through easy and affordable access to infertility treatments. In low-income countries, much infertility is caused by sexually transmitted and other infections as well as the complications from unsafe abortion. In poorer countries, involuntary primary infertility (i.e. the inability to bear any children) is often low compared to involuntary secondary infertility (i.e. the inability to have another child after having given birth to at least one).

Data from 47 developing countries (excluding China) show that in 2004 an estimated 187 million couples were affected by infertility – approximately 18 million with primary infertility and the remaining 169 million with secondary infertility. The percentage of couples with primary or secondary infertility was highest in countries of sub-Saharan Africa (30%) compared to countries in South-Central Asia (28%), South-East Asia (24%), and countries in Latin America and the Caribbean (16%).[29]

Figure 8 **Incidence rates of cervical cancer (age-standardized per 100 000 women, all ages), 2004**

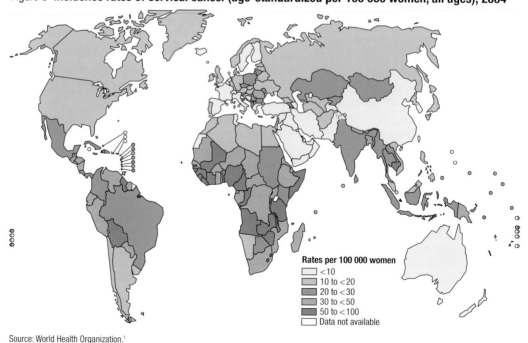

Rates per 100 000 women
- <10
- 10 to <20
- 20 to <30
- 30 to <50
- 50 to <100
- Data not available

Source: World Health Organization.[1]

Conclusion

This chapter has focused on many compelling issues relating to women's sexual and reproductive health. Chapter 5 shows how these issues should be considered in a wider discussion of the health of adult women – when they face many other health risks and challenges alongside those related specifically to sex and reproduction. Chapter 5 is therefore closely related to this one.

Summary findings and implications

■ Maternal health problems, including those resulting from unsafe abortion, are an important cause of death and disability among women, particularly in low-income settings, despite the fact that the interventions needed to prevent such problems are well known and cost-effective.

■ The leading cause of death of women of reproductive age in low- and middle-income countries is HIV/AIDS. Women are particularly vulnerable to infections for both biological and social reasons; they may be unable to obtain the knowledge they need to protect themselves or may not be in a position to use it. Tuberculosis is also a major cause of death among women in this age group.

■ Women in all parts of the world face a heavy burden of ill-health linked to sexually transmitted infections, including cervical cancer. Although many of these infections can be prevented and treated, women in many parts of the world have no access to appropriate information and services.

■ Priorities for action include: increasing the number of births attended by skilled birth attendants in all countries with high maternal mortality rates; ensuring that a continuum of antenatal, delivery and post-partum care is available and accessible to all pregnant women; and ensuring that all women have access to modern contraception, safe abortion services (to the fullest extent permitted by law) including post-abortion care, and screening and treatment for sexually transmitted infections, including HIV and HPV. Equally important are strategies to prevent and respond to intimate partner violence and sexual violence, and to empower women and increase their opportunities for participating in economic activities. It is vital to ensure that women have access to essential reproductive health care and services during humanitarian crises.

References

1. *The global burden of disease, 2004 update.* Geneva, World Health Organization, 2008.
2. *Global health risks: mortality and burden of disease attributable to selected major risks.* Geneva, World Health Organization (in press).
3. *Maternal mortality in 2005: estimates developed by WHO, UNICEF, UNFPA, and the World Bank.* Geneva, World Health Organization, 2007
4. *Tracking progress in maternal, newborn, and child survival. The 2008 report.* New York, NY, The United Nations Children's Fund (UNICEF), 2008.
5. ChildInfo: monitoring the situation of children and women, New York, NY, The United Nations Children's Fund (UNICEF), 2009 (http://www.childinfo.org, accessed 22 April 2009).
6. STAT compiler. Analysis of data from Demographic and Health Surveys published between 2003 and 2009. Calverton, MD, ICF Macro (http://www.measuredhs.com/).
7. Sedgh G et al. Induced abortion: estimated rates and trends worldwide. *Lancet*, 2007, 370:1338–1345. PMID:17933648 doi:10.1016/S0140-6736(07)61575-X
8. *The world health report, 2008 – primary health care: now more than ever.* Geneva, World Health Organization, 2008.
9. Westoff CF. *Recent trends in abortion and contraception in 12 countries.* DHS Analytical Studies, No 8. Calverton, MD, ORC Macro, 2005.

10. *World contraceptive use 2007.* New York, NY, United Nations, 2008.

11. *The Millennium Development Goals report.* New York, NY, United Nations, 2008.

12. Ribeiro PS, Jacobsen KH, Mathers CD, Garcia-Moreno C. Priorities for women's health from the Global Burden of Disease study. *International Journal of Gynaecology and Obstetrics: the Official Organ of the International Federation of Gynaecology and Obstetrics*, 2008, 102:82–90. PMID:18387613 doi:10.1016/j.ijgo.2008.01.025

13. Chersich MF, Rees HV. Vulnerability of women in southern Africa to infection with HIV: biological determinants and priority health sector interventions. *AIDS (London, England)*, 2008, 22 suppl 4;S27–S40. PMID:19033753doi:10.1097/01.aids.0000341775.94123.75

14. Preventing new HIV infections: the key to reversing the epidemic – Chapter 4. In: *2008 Report on the global AIDS epidemic.* Geneva, Joint United Nations Programme on HIV/AIDS (UNAIDS), 2008 (http://data.unaids.org/pub/GlobalReport/2008/jc1510_2008_global_report_pp95_128_en.pdf, accessed 18 July 2009).

15. *Towards universal access: scaling up priority HIV/AIDS interventions in the health sector: progress report 2008.* Geneva, World Health Organization, 2008 (http://www.who.int/hiv/pub/towards_universal_access_report_2008.pdf, accessed 26 June 2009).

16. Analysis of data from Demographic and Health Surveys in selected countries, 2005–2007. Calverton MD, Macro International Inc.

17. *HIV prevalence estimates from the Demographic and Health Surveys.* Calverton, MD, Macro International Inc., 2008.

18. *Strategies to support the HIV-related needs of refugees and host populations.* Geneva, Joint United Nations Programme on HIV/AIDS (UNAIDS) and United Nations High Commissioner for Refugees (UNHCR), 2005 (http://data.unaids.org/publications/IRC-pub06/jc1157-refugees_en.pdf, accessed 25 June 2005).

19. *Progress on implementing the Dublin Declaration on Partnership to Fight HIV/AIDS in Europe and Central Asia.* Copenhagen, WHO Regional Office for Europe and Joint United Nations Programme on HIV/AIDS (UNAIDS), 2008.

20. *2008 Report on the global AIDS epidemic.* Geneva, Joint United Nations Programme on HIV/AIDS (UNAIDS), 2008.

21. *HIV/AIDS prevention and care for female injecting drug users.* Vienna, United Nations Office on Drugs and Crime (UNODC), 2006 (http://www.unodc.org/pdf/HIV-AIDS_femaleIDUs_Aug06.pdf, accessed 18 July 2009).

22. *The global state of harm reduction 2008: mapping the response to drug-related HIV and Hepatitis C epidemics.* London, International Harm Reduction Association, 2008 (http://www.ihra.net/GlobalState2008, accessed 18 July 2009).

23. *At what cost? HIV and human rights consequences of the global "war on drugs".* New York, NY, Open Society Institute, 2008.

24. *Interventions to address HIV in prisons: HIV care, treatment and support.* Evidence for Action Technical Papers. Geneva, World Health Organization, 2007.

25. *HIV vulnerabilities of migrant women: from Asia to the Arab States.* Colombo, United Nations Development Regional Centre in Colombo, 2008 (http://www2.undprcc.lk/resource_centre/pub_pdfs/P1105.pdf, accessed 18 July 2009).

26. Glasier A et al. Sexual and reproductive health: a matter of life and death. *Lancet*, 2006, 368:1595–1607. PMID:17084760 doi:10.1016/S0140-6736(06)69478-6

27. Weinstock H, Berman S, Cates W Jr. Sexually transmitted diseases among American youth: incidence and prevalence estimates, 2000. *Perspectives on Sexual and Reproductive Health*, 2004, 36:6–10. PMID:14982671 doi:10.1363/3600604

28. Looker KJ, Garnett GP, Schmid GP. An estimate of the global prevalence and incidence of herpes simplex virus type 2 infection. *Bulletin of the World Health Organization*, 2008, 86:805–812. PMID:18949218 doi:10.2471/BLT.07.046128

29. Rutstein SO, Shah IH. *Infecundity, infertility, and childlessness in developing countries.* DHS Comparative Reports, No. 9. Calverton, MD, ORC Macro and the World Health Organization, 2004.

CHAPTER

5

ADULT WOMEN

Chapter 4 showed that sexual and reproductive health concerns are critically important for women around the world. This chapter shows that adult women face many other important health challenges, including chronic diseases, mental health, injuries and violence. This chapter looks at the health of women aged 20–59 years, here referred to as "adult women". Chapter 6 will focus on women aged 60 years and over, termed "older women".

Mortality and burden of disease

For women in developed countries, life between the ages of 20 and 60 years is generally a time of good health. There is a low risk of premature death - only 6% in high-income countries. Like their male counterparts, these adult women generally have a better life than their parents and grandparents did. Unfortunately, the situation is very different for hundreds of millions of women of comparable age in other parts of the world. In terms of the risk of premature death, the differences are stark. In the South-East Asia Region, for example, women face a 21% risk of death, and this proportion rises to 42% in the African Region. HIV/AIDS is by far the leading cause of death among adult women in Africa (Figure 1), but tuberculosis - often linked to HIV infection - is also a significant killer. Tuberculosis is also the second ranked cause of death in the Eastern Mediterranean and South-East Asia regions, and the fifth ranked cause of death for women in this age group worldwide (Table 1). In 2004, tuberculosis accounted for around 313 000 deaths among women aged 20–59 years.

While infectious diseases take a great toll, especially in Africa, it should be noted that half of the deaths among adult women globally are caused by noncommunicable diseases – particularly cardiovascular diseases, cancers and chronic respiratory diseases. As the health transition (described in Chapter 1) has progressed, noncommunicable diseases have become more significant and currently account for 80% of deaths among adult women in high-income countries, compared with only 25% in low-income countries. Injuries account for 15% of deaths globally among adult women, although there is considerable regional variation. Suicide and road traffic accidents are among the top 10 causes of death of adult women globally (Table 1).

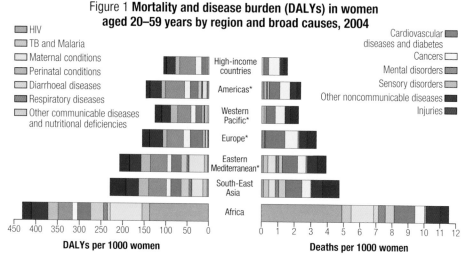

Figure 1 **Mortality and disease burden (DALYs) in women aged 20–59 years by region and broad causes, 2004**

HIV
TB and Malaria
Maternal conditions
Perinatal conditions
Diarrhoeal diseases
Respiratory diseases
Other communicable diseases and nutritional deficiencies

Cardiovascular diseases and diabetes
Cancers
Mental disorders
Sensory disorders
Other noncommunicable diseases
Injuries

High-income countries
Americas*
Western Pacific*
Europe*
Eastern Mediterranean*
South-East Asia
Africa

450 400 350 300 250 200 150 100 50 0
DALYs per 1000 women

0 1 2 3 4 5 6 7 8 9 10 11 12
Deaths per 1000 women

* High-income countries are excluded from the regional groups.
Source: World Health Organization.[1]

Mortality statistics alone do not capture the loss of health among adult women caused by chronic diseases, injuries and mental disorders, especially in developed countries. A better sense of the total burden of disease and injury suffered by women in this age group can be obtained by using DALYs (see Box 1 in Chapter 1). This alters the relative importance of different diseases, as can be seen in Figure 1. For example, cardiovascular diseases – mainly coronary heart disease and stroke (cerebrovascular disease) – killed 1.2 million women aged between 20 and 59 years in 2004 but caused ill-health and suffering to many millions more. Although it is sometimes assumed that these are the diseases of the richer countries, over 90% of them occur in low- and middle-income countries, which account for 85% of the world's women aged 20–59 years. Heart disease and stroke are the third and sixth leading causes of death in low-income countries.

In 2004, cancers killed just under one million women aged 20–59 years, with 80% of these deaths occurring in low- and middle-income countries, where women consistently have a lower cancer survival rate because of limited access to screening, late diagnosis, and inadequate access to effective treatment.[2,3] The most common cancer in women under age 60 globally is cancer of the breast, followed by cancers of the cervix, lung and stomach. Breast cancer is the leading cause of death among women between the ages of 20 and 59 years in high-income

Table 1 **Ten leading causes of death in women aged 20–59 years by country income group, 2004**

World				Low-income countries			
Rank	Cause	Deaths (000s)	%	Rank	Cause	Deaths (000s)	%
1	HIV/AIDS	835	13.3	1	HIV/AIDS	603	18.2
2	Maternal conditions	453	7.2	2	Maternal conditions	378	11.4
3	Ischaemic heart disease	429	6.8	3	Ischaemic heart disease	224	6.8
4	Stroke	360	5.7	4	Tuberculosis	213	6.4
5	Tuberculosis	313	5.0	5	Lower respiratory infections	138	4.2
6	Breast cancer	223	3.5	6	Stroke	128	3.9
7	Suicide	204	3.2	7	COPD*	90	2.7
8	Lower respiratory infections	190	3.0	8	Fires	88	2.7
9	Road traffic accidents	172	2.7	9	Suicide	77	2.3
10	COPD*	149	2.4	10	Cervical cancer	60	1.8

Middle-income countries				High-income countries			
Rank	Cause	Deaths (000s)	%	Rank	Cause	Deaths (000s)	%
1	HIV/AIDS	226	8.9	1	Breast cancer	49	11.5
2	Stroke	211	8.3	2	Trachea, bronchus, lung cancers	28	6.7
3	Ischaemic heart disease	177	6.9	3	Ischaemic heart disease	28	6.7
4	Breast cancer	116	4.6	4	Suicide	22	5.1
5	Suicide	104	4.1	5	Stroke	20	4.8
6	Road traffic accidents	102	4.0	6	Colon and rectum cancers	16	3.8
7	Tuberculosis	99	3.9	7	Road traffic accidents	16	3.8
8	Maternal conditions	74	2.9	8	Cirrhosis of the liver	13	3.1
9	Diabetes mellitus	65	2.5	9	Ovarian cancer	12	2.8
10	Cirrhosis of the liver	57	2.2	10	Cervical cancer	10	2.4

*Chronic obstructive pulmonary disease.
Source: World Health Organization.[1]

countries, where it causes more than one in every 10 deaths in this age group. Cancers and other chronic diseases are discussed further in the next chapter insofar as they affect older women.

Injuries are a leading cause of death and disability for adult women in all regions. The South-East Asia Region has a dispro-portionately high rate of fire-related deaths, while self-inflicted injuries are particularly high in developing countries of the Western Pacific Region (Figure 2). Road traffic acci-dents are relatively common in all regions and were responsible for an estimated 275 000 deaths of women aged 20–59 years in 2004.

Fire-related injuries are of particular concern to women since they suffer signifi-

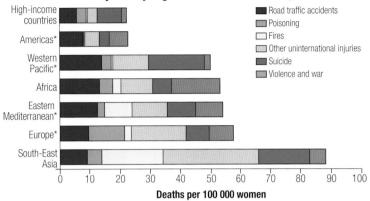

Figure 2 **Death rates due to injury in women aged 20–59 years by region and external causes, 2004**

* High-income countries are excluded from the regional groups.
Source: World Health Organization.[1]

cantly more of them than men do. Every year 168 000 adults aged 20–59 years worldwide die from unintentional fire-related injuries and 62% of them are women. A full 80% of these fire-related deaths happen in South-East Asia. Millions more women suffer burn-related disabilities and disfigurements, many of them permanent. These injuries can set off a cascade of second-ary personal and economic problems for both the victim and her family. Many fire deaths are probably related to cooking accidents but this is not the only cause. In India, fire is implicated in an estimated 16% of suicides in women and an unknown number of homicides.[4]

The health of women who live in poverty in countries that are themselves poor is severely affected by conditions that more well-off women around the world have never heard of. These conditions include 14 neglected tropical diseases that are found in over 100 of the poorest countries, particularly in Africa but also in Asia and Latin America. Most of the diseases can be prevented or eliminated altogether but many remain very common, affecting some 100 mil-lion people in total.

An estimated 56 million adult women have schistosomiasis. A further 28 million are infected with intestinal nematodes. Some 12 million have lymphoedema caused by lymphatic filiariasis. Adult women are three times more likely than men to develop the blinding compli-cation of trachoma because they are more likely to be infected through close contact with their children. This highly infectious disease, although completely preventable and treatable, blinds an estimated one million of the world's poorest women and is in the process of destroying the sight of others at a rate of between four and five million a year.

Women, depression and suicide

While women are less likely than men to suffer from alcohol and drug use disorders, they are more susceptible to depression and anxiety. An estimated 73 million adult women worldwide suffer a major depressive episode each year. Mental disorders following childbirth, includ-ing postpartum depression, are estimated to affect about 13% of women within one year of delivery.

Figure 3 **Percentage of people aged 20–59 years reporting moderate/severe mental disorders who received treatment, by sex and country income group, 21 selected countries, 2001–2007**

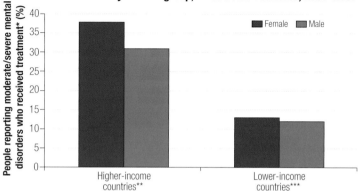

* Reported cases identified using standardized pre-defined algorithm based on DSM IV. Treatment was received during 12 months preceding the survey.
** High-income and upper middle-income countries.
*** Low-income and lower middle-income countries.
Source: World Mental Health Surveys in 21 countries, 2001–2007.[5]

In higher income[a] countries, almost 40% of women who report moderate or severe mental disorders received treatment during the previous 12 months, compared with only around 14% in lower income[b] countries (Figure 3). In both high- and low-income countries, women in the poorest households report more mental ill-health than women in the wealthiest ones and yet a smaller proportion of them receive treatment.[5] In high-income settings a smaller proportion of women with low education receive treatment compared with women with higher levels of education, but the reverse pattern is seen in low-income countries. Accompanying generally lower levels of treatment in low-income countries, the fact that women with higher levels of education in these settings are even less likely to receive care than those with low education suggests additional barriers to care. It is possible that stigma, associated with incorrect knowledge and negative attitudes, prevents access to care in addition to the limited availability of services.

Suicide, arguably the most extreme expression of mental illness, is the seventh leading cause of death globally for women aged 20–59 years, and the second leading cause of death in low- and middle-income countries of the Western Pacific Region. One in three female suicides worldwide occurs in women between 25 and 44 years of age. Suicide is the fifth leading cause of death globally for women aged 20–44 years, putting it ahead of road traffic accidents.

More women attempt suicide than men and suicidal behaviours are a significant public health problem for girls and women worldwide. The factors that increase the risk of suicide in women include exposure to childhood sexual abuse and intimate partner violence (discussed below). Abusive alcohol consumption is another risk factor, leading to depression and opening the way to intentional self-harm.[6] Gender differences in social roles may also play a part in suicidal behaviour. There is evidence in some cultures that social inequality and membership in tightly structured social units, especially patriarchal families, are risk factors for female suicidal behaviour. In China, where suicide is the leading cause of death among adult women in rural areas and where suicide rates of women are higher than those of men,[7] the most significant contributing factors are considered to be severe stress from acute life events and the ready availability of potentially lethal pesticides.

Risk factors for chronic disease

Much of the burden of disease that adult women face could be prevented by addressing critical risk factors. It is important to understand that each risk has specific causes.

Six risk factors for chronic disease jointly account for 37% of global deaths in women aged 30 years and over.[8] These risk factors account for 63% of deaths from cardiovascular disease and diabetes and over three-quarters of deaths from ischaemic heart disease. They are also

---

a Comprising high-income and higher middle-income countries according to the World Bank classification.
b Comprising low-income and lower middle-income countries according to the World Bank classification.

responsible for substantial numbers of women's deaths from cancer and chronic respiratory disease. While most of the deaths caused by these risk factors occur at older ages, much of the exposure starts earlier in life, often during adolescence, as mentioned in Chapter 3. Preventive interventions need to be targeted at younger women as much as, if not more than, at older women.

High blood pressure is the leading risk for adult women everywhere and is responsible for 18% of deaths of women over 20 years of age (Table 2) . High blood pressure, high blood glucose levels, physi-

Table 2 **Deaths in women aged 20 years and over attributable to six leading risk factors for chronic diseases, 2004 (percentage)**

Risk	World	Low-income countries	Middle-income countries	High-income countries
	Percentage of deaths			
High blood pressure	18	13	22	19
High blood glucose	8	8	8	7
Physical inactivity	8	6	8	8
Tobacco use	7	2	8	14
Overweight and obesity	7	4	9	9
High cholesterol	6	5	6	6

Source: World Health Organization.[8]

cal inactivity and high serum cholesterol cause similar proportions of deaths across all income levels. Tobacco smoking, overweight and obesity are currently more prevalent in middle- and high-income countries. That said, the incidence of these problems is rising in low- and middle-income countries. It is important to note that cost-effective interventions to address these major risk factors in adult women are available at population and individual levels.[9]

Tobacco use is one of the most serious avoidable risk factors for premature death and disease in adult women and is responsible for about 6% of female deaths worldwide.[8] Globally, 71% of lung cancer deaths are caused by tobacco use. Without continued action to reduce smoking, deaths among women aged 20 years and over will rise from 1.5 million in 2004 to 2.5 million by 2030; almost 75% of these projected deaths will occur in low- and middle-income countries.[8]

Tobacco and other environmental and behavioural risk factors are responsible for 35% of cancer deaths. Together with known infectious agents such as HPV and hepatitis B and C, these modifiable risk factors explain 42% of global cancer deaths in women aged 30 years and over. Tobacco is also implicated in about 42% of chronic respiratory disease and nearly 10% of cardiovascular disease in women.

Overweight and obesity are major risk factors for cardiovascular diseases, diabetes, musculoskeletal disorders and some cancers. Together they caused an estimated 1.5 million deaths in women aged 30 years and over in 2004, 77% of them in low- and middle-income countries. Many such countries are experiencing a rapid upsurge in chronic disease risk factors, particularly in urban settings. WHO's latest projections indicate that by 2015 the number of overweight and obese adult women will rise to 1.5 billion.

Violence

Violence against women is a widespread experience worldwide with serious public health implications. Violence against women can lead directly to serious injury, disability or death. It can also lead indirectly to a variety of health problems such as stress-induced physiological changes, substance use, or lack of fertility control and personal autonomy as often seen in abusive relationships. Abused women have higher rates of unintended pregnancies, abortions, adverse pregnancies and neonatal and infant outcomes, sexually transmitted infections (including HIV), and mental disorders (such as depression, anxiety disorders, sleep disorders and eating disorders)[10–17] compared to their non-abused peers.

Most violence against women is perpetrated by intimate male partners. A WHO study in 11 countries found that between 15% and 71% of women, depending on the country, had

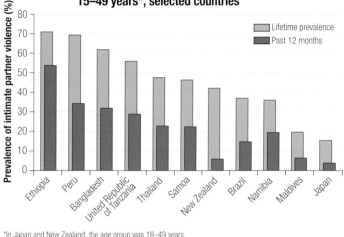

Figure 4 **Prevalence of physical or sexual violence, or both, by an intimate partner among women aged 15–49 years*, selected countries**

*In Japan and New Zealand, the age group was 18–49 years.
Note: Data drawn from specific provinces or cities, except for Maldives and Samoa.
Source: World Health Organization.[18]

experienced physical or sexual violence by a husband or partner in their lifetime, and 4% to 54% had experienced it within the previous year (Figure 4).[19] Partner violence may also be fatal. Studies from Australia, Canada, Israel, South Africa and the United States show that between 40% and 70% of female murders were carried out by intimate partners.[20] Sexual violence, whether by partners, acquaintances or strangers, also affects primarily women and girls. In conflict and post-conflict situations sexual violence is increasingly recognized as a tactic of war.

Other forms of violence against women include sexual harassment and abuse by authority figures (such as teachers, police officers or employers), trafficking for forced labour or sex, and traditional practices such as forced or child marriages and dowry-related violence. Violence against women is often related to social and gender bias and, at its most extreme, may lead to violent death or female infanticide. Despite the size of the problem, many women do not report their experiences of violence and do not seek help. As a result, violence against women remains a hidden problem with great human and health-care costs.

Illness and use of health services

Chronic conditions that require ongoing medical care – such as asthma, heart disease, arthritis, depression and diabetes – are common in women as they age, particularly in poorer women and those living in rural areas.[21] Most of these conditions can be prevented or managed effec-

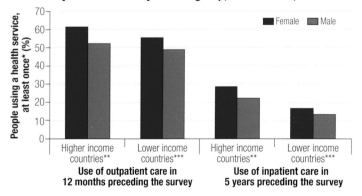

Figure 5 **Use of health-care services by people aged 20–59 years, by sex and country income group, 59 countries, 2002–2004**

* Service use by women for family planning, antenatal and delivery care is excluded.
** High-income and upper middle-income countries.
*** Low-income and lower middle-income countries.
Source: World Health Surveys in 59 countries, 2002–2004.

tively. Needed interventions include health education, control of risk factors, screening programmes, and access to cost-effective treatment.[1,22] Yet these are not available to many women. Although evidence is patchy and incomplete, it seems likely that there is a significant unmet need for medical care among women in lower income countries. While utilization rates of outpatient care are broadly similar around the world, there are major differences in inpatient utilization rates between women in lower income countries and those in higher income countries (Figure 5). The poorest women in lower income countries have utilization rates that are 50% lower than the wealthiest women in higher income countries.[22]

Conclusion

Adult women face a range of health challenges that include growing risks for chronic non-communicable diseases, injuries and violence. Suicide is one of the leading causes of death in women between the ages of 20 and 59 years globally and the second leading cause of death in the low- and middle-income countries of the Western Pacific Region. Mental health problems, particularly depression, are major causes of disability in women of all ages. Women's low status in society, their burden of work, and the violence they experience are all contributing factors. For many of these problems, effective interventions are available but progress in increasing access to the services that could make a difference to women's health is uneven. As women go through adulthood, those who are poor and live in rural areas face an unmet need for health-care services related to mental health and chronic conditions such as asthma, heart disease, arthritis and diabetes - all of which require ongoing medical care.

Summary findings and implications

■ Globally, rates of premature mortality in women aged 20–59 years are low. However, this is not the case in the African Region where more than two women in every five will die during this period of their lives, mostly from infectious diseases including HIV/AIDS.

■ As the health transition continues, deaths and disabilities in adult women are increasingly due to non-communicable diseases such as cardiovascular diseases, cancers, injuries and mental disorders, including suicide. Fire-related injuries are of particular concern to women in South-East Asia while suicide is a major cause of death and disability in the Western Pacific Region.

■ High blood pressure – often related to overweight, obesity and physical inactivity – is the leading risk factor for adult women. Violence is an important, though poorly measured, risk factor for a range of adverse health problems as well as being a direct cause of death and disability in women.

■ There is a need for health services to be organized so that they address the evolving needs of adult women. Currently, some services, such as antenatal care, are more likely to be in place than others – such as those related to mental health, chronic noncommunicable conditions and violence. Effective interventions include better access to health education, control of risk factors, implementation of screening programmes, and access to cost-effective treatment.

References

1. *The global burden of disease: 2004 update.* Geneva, World Health Organization, 2008.

2. Kamangar F, Dores GM, Anderson WF. Patterns of cancer incidence, mortality, and prevalence across five continents: defining priorities to reduce cancer disparities in different geographic regions of the world. *Journal of Clinical Oncology*, 2006, 24:2137–2150.doi:10.1200/JCO.2005.05.2308 PMID:16682732

3. Parkin DM, Bray F, Ferlay J, Pisani P. CA Global cancer statistics, 2002. *CA: a Cancer Journal for Clinicians*, 2005, 55:74–108.doi:10.3322/canjclin.55.2.74 PMID:15761078

4. Sanghavi P, Bhalla K, Das V. Fire-related deaths in India in 2001: a retrospective analysis of data. *Lancet*, 2009, 373:1282–1288.doi:10.1016/S0140-6736(09)60235-X PMID:19250664

5. Kessler RC, Ustun TB, eds. *The WHO World Mental Health Surveys: global perspectives on the epidemiology of mental disorders.* New York, NY, Cambridge University Press, 2008.

6. Rehm J et al. Alcohol use. In: Ezzati M, Lopez A, Rodgers A, Murray C, et al., eds. *Comparative quantification of health risks: global and regional burden of disease attributable to selected major risk factors.* Vol 1. Geneva, World Health Organization, 2004.

7. WHO mortality database. Geneva, World Health Organization (http://www.who.int/healthinfo/morttables/en/).

8. *Global health risks: mortality and burden of disease attributable to selected major risks.* Geneva, World Health Organization (in press).

9. Beaglehole R et al. Improving the prevention and management of chronic disease in low-income and middle-income countries: a priority for primary health care. *Lancet*, 2008, 372:940–949. doi:10.1016/S0140-6736(08)61404-X PMID:18790317

10. Campbell JC. Health consequences of intimate partner violence. *Lancet*, 2002, 359:1331–1336. doi:10.1016/S0140-6736(02)08336-8 PMID:11965295

11. Plichta SB, Falik M. Prevalence of violence and its implications for women's health. *Women's Health Issues*, 2001, 11:244–258.doi:10.1016/S1049-3867(01)00085-8 PMID:11336864

12. Dunkle KL et al. Gender-based violence, relationship power, and risk of HIV infection in women attending antenatal clinics in South Africa. *Lancet*, 2004, 363:1415–1421.doi:10.1016/S0140-6736(04)16098-4 PMID:15121402

13. Vos T et al. Measuring the impact of intimate partner violence on the health of women in Victoria, Australia. *Bulletin of the World Health Organization*, 2006, 84:739–744.doi:10.2471/BLT.06.030411 PMID:17128344

14. Campbell JC et al. The intersection of intimate partner violence against women and HIV/AIDS: a review. *International Journal of Injury Control and Safety Promotion*, 2008, 15:221–231. doi:10.1080/17457300802423224 PMID:19051085

15. Asling-Monemi K, Tabassum NR, Persson LA. Violence against women and the risk of under-five mortality: analysis of community-based data from rural Bangladesh. *Acta Paediatrica (Oslo, Norway: 1992)*, 2008, 97:226–232.doi:10.1111/j.1651-2227.2007.00597.x PMID:18254912

16. Ahmed S, Koenig MA, Stephenson R. Effects of domestic violence on perinatal and early-childhood mortality: evidence from north India. *American Journal of Public Health*, 2006, 96:1423–1428.doi:10.2105/AJPH.2005.066316 PMID:16809594

17. Boy A, Salihu HM. Intimate partner violence and birth outcomes: a systematic review. *International Journal of Fertility and Women's Medicine*, 2004, 49:159–164. PMID:15481481

18. Garcia-Moreno C et al. *WHO multi-country study on women's health and domestic violence. Initial results on prevalence, health outcomes and women's responses.* Geneva, World Health Organization, 2005.

19. Garcia-Moreno C et al. Prevalence of intimate partner violence: findings from the WHO multi-country study on women's health and domestic violence against women. *Lancet*, 2006, 368:1260–1269.doi:10.1016/S0140-6736(06)69523-8 PMID:17027732

20. Krug EG et al. *World report on violence and health.* Geneva, World Health Organization, 2002.

21. *World health survey.* World Health Organization. Geneva (http://www.who.int/healthinfo/survey/en/index.html, accessed 18 June 2009).

22. Jamison DT et al. *Disease control priorities in developing countries*, 2nd ed. New York, NY, Oxford University Press, 2006.

CHAPTER 6

OLDER WOMEN

Inevitably, mortality and disability rates rise at older ages but the extent and rapidity of these increases is not the same across all regions. While communicable diseases continue to take their toll in low-income settings, and particularly in Africa, the overall pattern of mortality and disability among women is characterized by a predominance of noncommunicable diseases, especially cardiovascular diseases (heart disease and stroke) as well as diabetes and cancers (Figure 1).

Women and ageing

Because they tend to live longer than men, women represent a growing proportion of all older people. Worldwide in 2007, 55% of adults aged 60 years and over were women, a proportion that rises to 58% at age 70 and above.[2] Ageing is sometimes assumed to be a concern mainly in countries with low birth rates, high incomes and effective geriatric health care. But in fact, the developing regions of the world are home to the majority of older women. In 2007, there were 270 million women aged 60 years and over living in low- and middle-income countries, compared with 115 million in high-income countries. The proportion of older people in the total population is increasing over time (Figure 2). By 2050, 84% of the population over age 60 is expected to be living in countries currently classified as low-income and middle-income.

Far from being a social or economic burden, this growing pool of older women should be viewed as a potential resource for society. For example, older women play key roles in their families and communities, acting as caregivers – including during humanitarian crises.[3] In countries with severe HIV epidemics, older women play a crucial role in caring for the large numbers of orphans. In 18 national surveys in sub-Saharan Africa, half of all orphans not living with a surviving parent were taken care of by grandparents, mostly the grandmother.[4]

Ways should be found to extend and enhance the lives these older women live. This is a twofold challenge which involves both taking action early on to prevent the development of chronic disease and providing health care specifically designed to manage the health problems women encounter as they age. Keeping older women healthy, fit and active not only benefits the individual but also makes sound economic and social sense; preventive interventions can help reduce the costs of long-term care for chronic conditions. However, this cannot be

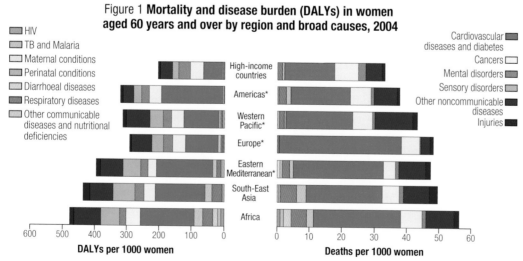

Figure 1 **Mortality and disease burden (DALYs) in women aged 60 years and over by region and broad causes, 2004**

* High-income countries are excluded from the regional groups.
Source: World Health Organization.[1]

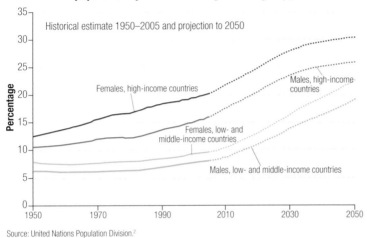

Figure 2 **Persons aged 60 years and over as a percentage of total population by sex and country income group, 1950–2050**

Historical estimate 1950–2005 and projection to 2050

Females, high-income countries

Males, high-income countries

Females, low- and middle-income countries

Males, low- and middle-income countries

Source: United Nations Population Division.[2]

achieved without significant forward planning and public health action. The challenges to health systems are particularly acute in high-income countries with low levels of fertility and growing proportions of older people in the population. But they are increasingly relevant in today's low- and middle-income countries where the trends identified above have emerged only recently and health systems remain largely geared to the health needs of younger women, especially those of reproductive age, and to the management of communicable diseases.

Socioeconomic influences on health in older women

The health of older women varies significantly from culture to culture and country to country. In many so-called "traditional" societies, for instance, where the extended family predominates, older women often acquire enhanced social status when their children marry and have their own children. However, increasing urbanization and more nuclear family structures often lead to isolation of the elderly of both sexes.

Because women tend to marry older men, and because women usually live longer, many older women will be widows. In most cases, they adjust both emotionally and financially to their changed situation. However, in some settings traditional practices relating to widowhood may result in violence and the abuse of older women, posing a serious threat to their health and well-being.[5]

In the few countries that have sound data on poverty levels by age and sex (mostly developed countries), there is evidence that older women are more likely to be poor than older men are.[6,7] Little is known about the extent to which women in developing countries face similar problems.

What are the health problems that older women face?

Globally, the leading causes of death and disability among women over age 60 are ischaemic heart disease, stroke and chronic obstructive pulmonary disease (Table 1). Together, these conditions account for 45% of deaths in women over 60 worldwide. A further 15% of deaths are caused by cancers – mainly cancers of the breast, lung and colon.

As with men, many of the health problems faced by women in old age are the result of risk factors experienced in their youth and adulthood. Smoking, sedentary lifestyles, and diets that are heavy in cholesterol, saturated fat and salt, but low in fresh fruits and vegetables, all contribute to the health problems women experience later in life.

Cardiovascular disease, often thought to be a "male" problem, is the main killer of older people of *both* sexes almost everywhere in the world. In fact, each year cardiovascular disease causes a larger number of deaths in older women than in older men – 7.4 million women over 60 years of age compared to 6.3 million men in 2004.[1] Although cardiovascular diseases are often thought of as diseases of affluence, cardiovascular mortality rates for women age 60 and over are more than twice as high in low- and middle-income countries as in high-income countries. They are particularly high in middle-income European countries, followed by the Eastern Mediterranean and the African regions.[1]

Part of the explanation is that cardiovascular mortality rates among women in high-income countries have significantly declined over the past 50 years (Figure 3). These declines are the result of several factors, namely: reductions in risk behaviours such as use of tobacco and lack of physical activity; better management and medication of metabolic risk factors such as high blood pressure and high cholesterol; and improved treatment of existing cardiovascular conditions.[8]

There is no reason why the same declines should not be achieved in middle-income countries today, but the necessary public health interventions have yet to be widely implemented. Meanwhile, access to cost-effective pharmaceutical interventions is lacking, as is the prompt treatment of cardiovascular conditions to improve survival.

Cardiovascular disease in women is often unrecognized, especially in low- and middle-income countries, for a number of reasons. Women with acute coronary syndromes often

Table 1 **Ten leading causes of death in women aged 60 years and over by country income group, 2004**

World				Low-income countries			
Rank	Cause	Deaths (000s)	%	Rank	Cause	Deaths (000s)	%
1	Ischaemic heart disease	2933	19.2	1	Ischaemic heart disease	829	19.9
2	Stroke	2677	17.5	2	Stroke	613	14.7
3	COPD*	1254	8.2	3	Lower respiratory infections	403	9.7
4	Lower respiratory infections	818	5.3	4	COPD*	313	7.5
5	Diabetes mellitus	499	3.3	5	Diabetes mellitus	143	3.4
6	Hypertensive heart disease	453	3.0	6	Hypertensive heart disease	89	2.1
7	Alzheimer and other dementias	305	2.0	7	Cervical cancer	78	1.9
8	Breast cancer	294	1.9	8	Nephritis and nephrosis	73	1.8
9	Trachea, bronchus and lung cancers	287	1.9	9	Diarrhoeal diseases	71	1.7
10	Colon and rectum cancers	241	1.6	10	Breast cancer	64	1.5

Middle-income countries				High-income countries			
Rank	Cause	Deaths (000s)	%	Rank	Cause	Deaths (000s)	%
1	Stroke	1625	21.7	1	Ischaemic heart disease	622	17.1
2	Ischaemic heart disease	1481	19.8	2	Stroke	438	12.1
3	COPD*	821	11.0	3	Alzheimer and other dementias	194	5.3
4	Hypertensive heart disease	278	3.7	4	Lower respiratory infections	158	4.4
5	Lower respiratory infections	256	3.4	5	Trachea, bronchus and lung cancers	130	3.6
6	Diabetes mellitus	242	3.2	6	COPD*	120	3.3
7	Stomach cancer	145	1.9	7	Breast cancer	114	3.1
8	Trachea, bronchus and lung cancers	136	1.8	8	Colon and rectum cancers	114	3.1
9	Breast cancer	115	1.5	9	Diabetes mellitus	113	3.1
10	Colon and rectum cancers	106	1.4	10	Hypertensive heart disease	86	2.4

*Chronic obstructive pulmonary disease.
Source: World Health Organization.[1]

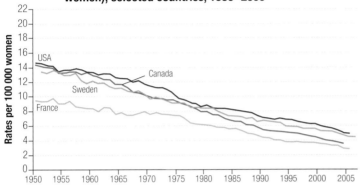

Figure 3 **Mortality rates due to cardiovascular diseases in women aged 30 years and over (age-standardized per 100 000 women), selected countries, 1950–2006**

Sources: WHO mortality database as of March 2009 (http://www.who.int/healthinfo/morttables/en/index.html); and United Nations Population Division.[2]

remain undiagnosed, in part because they often show different symptoms from men.[9–12] Women are also less likely than men to seek medical help, and therefore do not get appropriate care until later when urgent intervention is necessary but less likely to be successful.[13] Data from the World Health Surveys found that almost half of women in high-income and upper middle-income countries were receiving treatment for symptoms of chronic heart disease, compared with only one in four in low-income and lower middle-income countries.[14] Women also tend to develop heart disease later than men. This further complicates diagnosis because it means that other diseases, including diabetes and hypertension, are more likely to be present.[13] Unfortunately, women tend to be under-represented in mixed-sex clinical trials for heart disease treatments.[15] This has hampered development of sex-specific treatment guidelines.

Another leading cause of disease and death among older women is chronic obstructive pulmonary disease, or COPD. One of the main causes of COPD worldwide is tobacco use, an addiction that is often acquired at younger ages. But, as noted in Chapter 1, exposure to indoor air pollution caused by the burning of solid fuels for indoor heating and cooking is the primary risk factor for COPD in women. These exposures contribute to higher COPD mortality rates for older women in low- and middle-income countries, where rates are over five times higher than in high-income countries.[1,16]

The most common forms of cancer suffered by women are cancer of the breast, cervix and colon.[1] In terms of mortality, the biggest killers are breast, lung, colon and stomach cancer. Although these cancers can occur before the age of 60 years, most of the deaths (68%) occur at older ages. As might be expected, there are significant variations between countries in both cancer incidence and cancer types. This is also true of diagnosis and survival rates. For some cancers, such as lung cancer and colorectal cancer, both incidence (new cases) and mortality are higher in high-income countries. The reverse is true for cervical cancer, where incidence and mortality are higher in low-income countries (Figure 4).[1] This is mainly because of a higher incidence of HPV infection at younger ages. In addition, most women in high-income countries undergo screening for cervical cancer, thus increasing the chance of early diagnosis, which in turn improves the likelihood of effective treatment. By contrast, in low- and middle-income countries, women are more likely to die because of late detection and inadequate access to treatment.[17]

Incidence of breast cancer is considerably higher in high-income countries compared with low- and middle-income

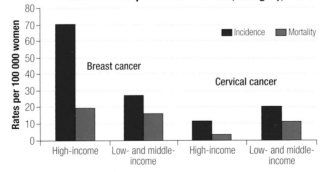

Figure 4 **Incidence and mortality rates of breast cancer and cervical cancer by country income group (age-standardized per 100 000 women, all ages), 2004**

Source: World Health Organization.[1]

countries, but mortality is similar (Figure 4). This is due to the availability of better treatment in the former countries. Early detection is essential for successful cancer treatment but data from several low-income countries suggest that mammography screening rates may be as low as 5% or less.[18] Detection needs to be accompanied by effective treatment of the cases identified. Unfortunately, for most women in many low- and middle-income countries, effective treatment is out of reach because it is unavailable, inaccessible or unaffordable.

Managing disabilities – a matter of prevention and care

One of the keys to an old age characterized by good health is healthy behaviour, preferably adopted early on in life – including healthy dietary choices and regular physical activity. Healthy behaviour can increase life expectancy and delay the onset of chronic conditions and disability, compressing the time spent in ill-health into a shorter period at the end of life.[19]

Despite this, ageing is often accompanied by declining health, including loss of muscular and cognitive functions, which can have far-reaching consequences. Ageing is also associated with increasing levels of comorbidity – i.e. when a person has several diseases or disabilities at the same time – which significantly complicates treatment. Data on the prevalence of disabling conditions are usually collected without considering this clustering of diseases. The main chronic and debilitating health problems faced by older women are poor vision (including cataracts), hearing loss, arthritis, depression and dementia (Table 2).

Some recent studies have found evidence that self-reported disability prevalence may be declining at all levels of severity in older adults in some developed countries.[20-24] Changing attitudes and increased acceptance of disability may have played a role in these declines. Nevertheless, the overall prevalence and severity of disability among older women will continue to increase due to the ageing of the population, and because higher proportions of older women will be in the oldest age groups where disability levels are higher.

Loss of vision causes 32% of total years lost due to disability[a] in women over the age of 60 years. Older women are not only more likely to suffer from blindness than older men, but they also face more difficulty in getting the care they need.[1] Across all ages, 57% of blind people in the world are female and this proportion rises with age. Why is this? In part, it is because women are not getting access to treatment.

Women over the age of 60 in low-income countries are nine times more likely to be blind than women in high-income countries, primarily due to cataracts and uncorrected refractive errors.[1] Worldwide, 44% of blindness among women over age 60 is caused by cataracts, which can be cured by simple and relatively cheap surgery.[1] Yet women with cataracts are less likely to have

Table 2 **Years lost due to disability (YLDs) among women aged 60 years and over by leading causes, 2004**

Disability	Low-income countries	Middle-income countries	High-income countries
	Millions of YLDs		
Alzheimer and other dementias	0.6 ▪	2.1 ▅	2.3 ▅
Refractive errors	2.0 ▆	1.6 ▅	0.5 ▪
Hearing loss, adult onset	1.0 ▪	1.6 ▅	1.0 ▪
Cataracts	1.3 ▪	1.9 ▅	0.1 ▏
Osteoarthritis	0.5 ▪	1.2 ▪	0.9 ▪
Unipolar depressive disorders	0.6 ▪	1.1 ▪	0.5 ▪
Macular degeneration	0.6 ▪	1.0 ▪	0.4 ▪
Ischaemic heart disease	0.4 ▪	0.7 ▪	0.3 ▪
Diabetes mellitus	0.1 ▏	0.6 ▪	0.4 ▪
Stroke	0.2 ▪	0.7 ▪	0.3 ▪

Source: World Health Organization.[1]

---

a YLDs, or years lost due to disability, are calculated as: the number of incident cases × average duration of the disease × weight factor to account for severity (http://www.who.int/healthinfo/global_burden_disease/GBD_report_2004update_part1.pdf).

cataract surgery than men because of the barriers to care that exist at both the family and community levels and because of an inadequate supply of services.[25]

Trachoma causes about 5% of blindness in low-income countries and yet is entirely preventable. Trachoma is more common in women because it is a highly infectious disease that is frequently passed from child to child and from child to mother, especially where water is in short supply, flies are numerous, and living conditions are crowded.[1]

Arthritis is another major cause of disability, with older people particularly at risk, notably to osteoarthritis and rheumatoid arthritis.[1] Overweight, which has become more prevalent in women than in men, is an important risk factor for osteoarthritis and is responsible for approximately 19% of cases among women aged over 60 years.[16] However, there seem to be few differences in prevalence across income groups, in rural and urban areas, and in low- and middle-income countries.[14] Although treatments are available to alleviate the suffering associated with arthritis, the available evidence indicates that only a minority of both women and men are receiving such care.

Osteoporosis is three times more common in women than in men.[26] Osteoporosis is a major risk factor for hip fractures, of which there were approximately 1.6 million worldwide in 2000.[27] Nearly 70% of these fractures occurred among women. Hip fractures cause substantial disability and often result in long-term institutionalization. In the United States, for example, about 20% of hip fracture patients require long-term care in a nursing home.[28]

Each year in developed countries, more than a third of people over the age of 70 years report falling.[29] Women are more likely to be injured in a fall, in part because of the higher prevalence of osteoporosis. Maintaining an active lifestyle is one of the most cost-effective ways to prevent falls and their consequences.[30]

Perhaps one of the greatest challenges faced by the individual woman as she ages, and by the society which surrounds her, is the disintegration of the self that occurs with dementia.

Dementia causes 13% of years of healthy life lost among women over 60 years of age. Women with dementia also face an increased risk of depression and require substantial resources for care. The prevalence of dementia appears to double approximately every five years after the age of 65 years. Older people who have a form of dementia as their main clinical condition are more likely to have severe restrictions on their activities. Assuming that age-specific dementia prevalence rates remain constant, the ageing of populations in many developed countries will result in a doubling in the prevalence of dementia by 2030 at the same time as death rates decline.

Caring for older women

With adequate health care and a supportive environment, women can remain active and healthy well into old age. However, health-care provision, especially in low- and middle-income countries and in times of humanitarian crisis, may be biased against the old and is rarely geared to the particular needs of older women. In many countries, access to health care is dependent on social security and health insurance systems, which in turn are linked to previous employment in the formal sector of the economy. Because many older women in developing countries work all of their lives in the informal sector or in unpaid activities, health care is inaccessible, unaffordable or both.

In many settings, especially in developing countries, the care of older people is often provided informally by family and neighbours, and falls primarily on the female family members.[31] The provision of that care imposes significant economic, social and health burdens on the caregivers,[31] including a higher risk of depression. In high-income countries, care of the elderly may be covered by social insurance schemes but mounting costs mean that family members often have to make substantial financial contributions to such care. Studies in Estonia, Latvia and Uganda, for example, show that households with members over 65 years of age are more likely to face catastrophic health expenditure than households with no elderly members.[32-34]

As the number of older people continues to increase compared to the pool of available caregivers, and as traditional social structures break down, families and policy-makers will increasingly need to look for other options. The situation is exacerbated in many rural areas of developing countries where the migration of younger people to cities has left many older women without family support. Part of the answer may lie in increased home and community support services, but it is likely that the number of very old women who spend their last years in institutional settings will also increase.[35]

Unfortunately, the stresses associated with long-term care, whether in the home or in an institutional setting, may be associated with neglect and abuse of elderly women. Until very recently, the abuse of older people was a social problem hidden from public view. Evidence is accumulating, however, that elder abuse – which includes both harmful actions and lack of action – is an important public health and societal problem that manifests itself in both developing and developed countries.[36]

Conclusion

Chronic conditions – ischaemic heart disease, stroke and chronic obstructive pulmonary disease – account for 45% of deaths in women over 60 years of age worldwide. A further 15% of deaths are caused by cancers, mainly of the breast, lung and colon. Many of the health problems faced by women in old age are the result of risk factors that arise in their youth and adulthood – such as smoking, sedentary lifestyles, and unhealthy diets. Societies need to prepare now to prevent and manage the chronic health problems associated with old age. Establishing healthy habits at younger ages can help women to live active and healthy lives until well into old age. Societies must also prepare for the costs associated with the care of older women. Many high-income countries currently direct large proportions of their social and health budgets to care for the elderly. In low-income settings, such care is often the responsibility of the family, and usually of its female members. Policies are needed in relation to health financing, pension and tax reform, access to formal employment and associated pension and social protection, and the provision of residential and community care.

Summary findings and implications

■ The leading causes of death and disability among women over age 60 are ischaemic heart disease, stroke, chronic obstructive pulmonary disease and cancers. Many of the health problems faced by women in old age are the result of behaviours established in their youth and adulthood, including smoking, sedentary lifestyles, and diets heavy in cholesterol, saturated fat and salt, but low in fresh fruits and vegetables.

■ A major cause of disability in older women is vision loss; every year, more than 2.5 million older women go blind. Much of this burden of disability could be avoided if these women had access to the necessary care, particularly surgery for cataracts. However, women face difficulty in getting the care they need. In low-income countries, trachoma is a significant but preventable cause of blindness that affects women in particular.

■ With adequate health care and a supportive environment – including increasing opportunities for older women to contribute productively to society – women can remain active and healthy well into old age. However, in low- and middle-income countries, health care may be inaccessible due to cost and is rarely geared to the particular needs of older women.

■ Interventions should focus on promoting behavioural and lifestyle changes – such as healthy nutritional practices and active living. These can help prevent or delay some health problems. In ensuring access to care, there is a need for screening and treatment programmes for diabetes, cancer, hypertension and heart disease, as well as cataract repair services for women with low incomes.

■ It is essential to build "age-friendly environments" for older women. They need to be supported in their caring and other roles where needed. Longer and healthier life is a social goal that will give women opportunities that they and their communities will value, and at the same time will lead to major social changes in the organization of work, family and social support.

References

1. *The global burden of disease: 2004 update.* Geneva, World Health Organization, 2008.

2. *World population prospects. The 2006 revision.* New York, NY, United Nations Population Division, 2007.

3. *Humanitarian action and older persons. An essential brief for humanitarian actors.* Geneva, Inter-Agency Standing Committee, 2008.

4. Monasch R, Boerma JT. Orphanhood and childcare patterns:an analysis of national surveys from 40 countries. *AIDS (London, England),* 2004, 18 suppl 2;S55–S65.doi:10.1097/00002030-200406002-00007 PMID:15319744

5. Chen MA. *Perpetual mourning: widowhood in rural India.* Oxford, Oxford University Press, 2000.

6. Munnell AH. *Why are so many older women poor?* Working Paper No. 10. Chestnut Hill, MA, Boston College Center for Retirement Research, 2004 (http://ssrn.com/abstract=556788).

7. Houser AN. *Women and long-term care: research report.* Washington, DC, AARP, 2007 (http://www.aarp.org/research/longtermcare/trends/fs77r_ltc.html, accessed 18 July 2009).

8. Ford ES et al. Capewell, Simon Explaining the Decrease in U.S. Deaths from Coronary Disease, 1980-2000. *The New England Journal of Medicine,* 2007, 356:2388–2398.doi:10.1056/NEJMsa053935 PMID:17554120

9. Baumhäkel M, Müller U, Böhm M. Influence of gender of physicians and patients on guideline-recommended treatment of chronic heart failure in a cross-sectional study. *European Journal of Heart Failure,* 2009, 11:299–303.doi:10.1093/eurjhf/hfn041 PMID:19158153

10. Adams A et al. The influence of patient and doctor gender on diagnosing coronary heart disease. *Sociology of Health & Illness,* 2008, 30:1–18.doi:10.1111/j.1467-9566.2007.01025.x PMID:18254830

11. Hochman JS et al. Sex, clinical presentation, and outcome in patients with acute coronary syndromes. *The New England Journal of Medicine,* 1999, 341:226–232.doi:10.1056/NEJM199907223410402 PMID:10413734

12. Jneid H, Thacker HL. Coronary artery disease in women: different, often undertreated. *Cleveland Clinic Journal of Medicine,* 2001, 68:441–448.doi:10.3949/ccjm.68.5.441 PMID:11352324

13. Mikhail GW. Coronary heart disease in women. *BMJ (Clinical Research Ed.),* 2005, 331:467–468. doi:10.1136/bmj.331.7515.467 PMID:16141136

14. *World health survey.* Geneva, World Health Organization (http://www.who.int/healthinfo/survey/en/, accessed 18 June 2009).

15. Kim ESH, Carrigan TP, Menon V. Enrollment of women in National Heart, Lung, and Blood Institute-funded cardiovascular randomized controlled trials fails to meet current federal mandates for inclusion. *Journal of the American College of Cardiology,* 2008, 52:672–673. doi:10.1016/j.jacc.2008.05.025 PMID:18702973

16. *Global health risks: mortality and burden of disease attributable to selected major risks.* Geneva, World Health Organization (in press).

17. Gakidou E, Nordhagen S, Obermeyer Z. Coverage of cervical cancer screening in 57 countries: low average levels and large inequalities. *PLoS Medicine,* 2008, 5:e132.doi:10.1371/journal.pmed.0050132 PMID:18563963

18. *World health statistics 2008.* Geneva, World Health Organization, 2008.

19. Vita AJ, Terry RB, Hubert HB, Fries JF. Aging, health risks and cumulative disability. *The New England Journal of Medicine,* 1998, 338:1035–1041.doi:10.1056/NEJM199804093381506 PMID:9535669

20. Manton KG, Corder L, Stallard E. Chronic disability trends in elderly United States populations: 1982–1994. *Proceedings of the National Academy of Sciences of the United States of America,* 1997, 94:2593–2598.doi:10.1073/pnas.94.6.2593 PMID:9122240

21. Manton KG, Gu X. Changes in the prevalence of chronic disability in the United States black and nonblack population above age 65 from 1982 to 1999. *Proceedings of the National Academy of Sciences of the United States of America,* 2001, 98:6354–6359.doi:10.1073/pnas.111152298 PMID:11344275

22. Freedman VA, Martin LG. Understanding trends in functional limitations among older Americans. *American Journal of Public Health*, 1998, 88:1457–1462.doi:10.2105/AJPH.88.10.1457 PMID:9772844

23. Crimmins EM, Reynolds SL, Saito Y. Trends in health and ability to work among the older working-age population. *The Journals of Gerontology. Series B, Psychological Sciences and Social Sciences*, 1999, 54:S31–S40. PMID:9934400

24. Spiers N, Jagger C, Clarke M. Physical function and perceived health: cohort differences and interrelationships in older people. *The Journals of Gerontology. Series B, Psychological Sciences and Social Sciences*, 1996, 51:S226–S233.PMID:8809007

25. Lewallen S, Courtright P. Gender and use of cataract surgical services in developing countries. *Bulletin of the World Health Organization*, 2002, 80:300–303. PMID:12075366

26. *Prevention and management of osteoporosis.* WHO Technical Report Series, No 921. Geneva, World Health Organization, 2003.

27. Johnell O, Kanis JA. An estimate of the worldwide prevalence and disability associated with osteoporotic fractures. *Osteoporosis International*, 2006, 17:1726–1733.doi:10.1007/s00198-006-0172-4 PMID:16983459

28. Chrischilles E, Shireman T, Wallace R. Cost and health effects of osteoporosis fractures. *Bone*, 1994, 15:377–386.doi:10.1016/8756-3282(94)90813-3 PMID:7917575

29. *WHO global report on falls prevention in older age.* Geneva, World Health Organization, 2007.

30. Beard J et al. Economic analysis of a community-based falls prevention program. *Public Health*, 2006, 120:742–751.doi:10.1016/j.puhe.2006.04.011 PMID:16824563

31. Prince M. 10/66 Dementia Research Group. Care arrangements for people with dementia in developing countries. *International Journal of Geriatric Psychiatry*, 2004, 19:170–177.doi:10.1002/gps.1059 PMID:14758582

32. Xu K et al. Understanding the impact of eliminating user fees: Utilization and catastrophic health expenditures in Uganda. *Social Science & Medicine*, 2006, 62:866–876.doi:10.1016/j.socscimed.2005.07.004 PMID:16139936

33. Habicht J, Xu K, Couffinhal A, Kutzin J. Detecting changes in financial protection: creating evidence for policy in Estonia. *Health Policy and Planning*, 2006, 21:421–431.doi:10.1093/heapol/czl026 PMID:16951417

34. Xu K et al. *Access to health care and the financial burden of out-of-pocket health payments in Latvia.* Technical Brief for Policy-Makers, No 1/2009. Geneva, World Health Organization, 2009.

35. *Women, ageing and health: a framework for action.* Geneva, World Health Organization, 2007.

36. *A global response to elder abuse and neglect: building primary health care capacity to deal with the problem worldwide: main report.* Geneva, World Health Organization, 2008 (http://www.who.int/ageing/publications/ELDER_DocAugust08.pdf, accessed 18 July 2009).

CHAPTER 7

POLICY IMPLICATIONS

This final chapter considers the policy implications of the evidence presented in Chapters 1 to 6. It identifies opportunities for making more rapid progress, as well as areas in which further information – and policy dialogue at national, regional and international levels – could lead to more effective approaches and better outcomes for women's health.

Despite huge advances in health in recent years, women in many parts of the world still face health problems that should have been tackled many years ago. Elsewhere, women have benefited from progress only to find themselves confronting new problems, many of them chronic and emerging at older ages. These problems can be improved by health promotion and health-care interventions earlier in life.

Women and men share the same right to the enjoyment of the highest attainable standard of physical and mental health.[1] However, women are disadvantaged due to social, cultural, political and economic factors that directly influence their health and impede their access to health-related information and care. Strategies to improve women's health must take full account of the underlying determinants of health – particularly gender inequality – and must address the specific socioeconomic and cultural barriers that hamper women in protecting and improving their health. These strategies must be placed in the broader context of revitalized primary health care, which addresses both priority health needs and the underlying determinants of health.[2] Primary health care can make a difference through policy action to strengthen leadership, build responsive health services, achieve universal coverage and leverage change in public policy.

Leadership

Building strong leadership

Leadership is needed to make sure that all women reach their full health potential. The significant advances made in women's health in some countries indicate that it can be done. The interventions are known and the resources are attainable.

The lack of progress in some countries can partly be attributed to socioeconomic constraints, along with political instability, civil strife and other crises. However, differences in health status are also related to policy decisions and investments in key programme areas. It is important to recognize that health systems may not balance different programme areas effectively. Nor do they naturally lead to more equitable health outcomes. In fact, the trend is towards a widening gap in key health outcomes related to women's health, both between countries and within countries.

The Millennium Development Goals have been vitally important in providing impetus to accelerate action towards health goals within the context of development despite many other competing claims on the world's attention. The existence of a separate goal on maternal mortality draws attention to the lack of progress in this area, and has attracted both political and financial support for accelerating change. The addition of the target on universal access to reproductive health, in line with previous commitments on women's health,[a] has helped to broaden the scope of the goal. However, the focus remains limited to one aspect of women's lives, albeit a critical one. There is now a need to extend attention to the many other challenges to, and determinants of, women's health described in this report. In doing so, it is important to work towards gender equality and women's empowerment (Goal 3).

---

a For international commitments on women's health, see the Programme of Action adopted at the International Conference on Population and Development (ICPD), Cairo, 5–13 September 1994 (http://www.un.org/popin/icpd/conference/offeng/poa.html); and also the Beijing Declaration and Platform for Action of the Fourth World Conference on Women, 15 September 1995.

The situation is made more complex by the way women's health is handled both within and between international organizations, with multiple initiatives competing for attention and resources. National responses to women's health issues also tend to be fragmented and limited in scope. There is a need for sustained commitment to achieving results and for agreement on a coherent and unified approach.

Bold, participatory leadership with a clear and coherent agenda for action is key to moving forward. Leadership must take into account the range of issues that affect women's lives and must deliberately address problem areas where progress is inadequate or inequities are growing. The participation of civil society, and particularly women's health advocates and leaders, is critical. Their meaningful engagement at all levels of assessment, priority setting and implementation should be championed and their ability to bring decision-makers to account strengthened.

The role of gender mainstreaming

Over the past few years, "gender mainstreaming"[a] has become a preferred approach for achieving women's health. It stems from recognition that while technical strategies are necessary, they are not sufficient unless we address the gender discrimination, bias and inequality that permeate the organizational structures of governments and organizations – including health systems – and unless we change the way such structures operate ("institutional mainstreaming"). Gender mainstreaming also implies that gender concerns must be dealt with in every aspect of policy development and programming, through systematic gender analyses and the implementation of actions that address the balance of power and the distribution of resources between women and men ("operational mainstreaming").[3]

Gender mainstreaming in health aims to promote equality between women and men throughout the life course and to achieve health equity. The Women and Gender Equity Knowledge Network of the WHO Commission on Social Determinants of Health proposes concrete approaches to gender mainstreaming for health in government and nongovernmental organizations and describes collaborative efforts to protect the rights and health of women.[4,5] Documented experiences include many initiatives that are intended to address neglected issues and improve health outcomes for women. These initiatives range from efforts to press for breast and cervical cancer screening and treatment services in Ghana to the development of policies on abortion and violence against women in South Africa. Women leaders, including those in ministries of health, have a clear influence in driving these changes. In addition, efforts have been made to integrate gender into the training curricula of health professionals.[6,7]

To move beyond "business as usual" and to accelerate the pace of reform, some countries have taken deliberate steps to integrate gender analysis and actions into their public health policies. For instance, Sweden's public health policy specifically highlights its commitment to reducing gender-based inequities in health, alongside reductions in inequities by socioeconomic and ethnic group and geographical region.[8]

---

a Gender mainstreaming was defined by the United Nations Economic and Social Council in 1997 as follows: "Mainstreaming a gender perspective is the process of assessing the implications for women and men of any planned action, including legislation, policies or programmes, in all areas and at all levels. It is a strategy for making women's as well as men's concerns and experiences an integral dimension of the design, implementation, monitoring and evaluation of policies and programmes in all political, economic and societal spheres so that women and men benefit equally and inequality is not perpetuated. The ultimate aim is to achieve gender equality."

Building accountability

The focus on governance and the policy environment requires improved understanding and tracking of change in these areas. A useful example is provided by the Countdown to 2015 initiative which is promoting the use of indicators of health policies and health systems as critical complements to tracking coverage of interventions for the improvement of maternal, newborn and child health. The initiative proposes selected indicators to assess specific policies in relation to evidence and information, governance and leadership, quality and efficiency of care, financing of health services, and health workforce availability. Available data are provided for 68 priority countries.[9] Further work of this kind would help health leaders and governments identify the steps that must be taken to remove policy and health system impediments to progress, and to support the development of more effective accountability systems.

Some countries have taken steps to institutionalize such accountability systems. South Africa, for instance, not only requires that all maternal deaths be notified but also conducts audits of maternal deaths under an audit system called "every death counts" which also covers stillbirths, and neonatal and child deaths.[10]

Murthy has identified several mechanisms by which governments have promoted accountability on health, including women's health, to citizens.[11] Health observatories can serve this purpose, as they involve a range of stakeholders in tracking and interpreting data, with direct links to policy-making and to the sharing of best practices. In Latin America and elsewhere, there are several instances of health observatories being set up to bring together better data and to build accountability in order to reduce gender-based inequities in health. Some are run by civil society and others by ministries of women's affairs (as in Chile and Colombia), or ministries of health (as in Spain).[12] Some observatories are run by a combination of ministries, as is the case for observatories of gender-based violence in several countries.

Responsive health services

Health systems reflect the societies that create them. To avoid a situation where they contribute to perpetuating health inequities, they must become more responsive to the needs and expectations of women as both consumers and producers of health care.

What women need

A central tenet of primary health care is to "put people first".[2] This requires attention to specific features of health systems that are essential for improving health and social outcomes for women.

The first set of features addresses the responsiveness of the health services to women's health needs. Although women are the main users of health care, insufficient attention is given to their needs and perspectives throughout the life course, and to the constraints that they face in protecting their health or in accessing or making the most of available services. Key concerns for women seeking health care include respect, trust, privacy and confidentiality - values that are often compromised in busy facilities, particularly among certain age groups and social groups.[13]

Those responsible for health care are also responsible for protecting women's autonomy in respect of their own health. This means eliminating gender biases and discrimination in health services, and making sure that women are not excluded from services. For example, unmarried girls seeking care for sexually transmitted infections should receive that care, yet they are often ostracised while their male peers are able to access treatment. Women should not be refused contraception or other services if they do not have their partner's consent.[7] Further, health-care providers need to take firm action and speak out against practices that violate the rights and harm the health of women and girls – as with intimate partner violence, sexual violence, female genital mutilation, early marriage and other harmful practices.

Second, health systems must build capacity to address the broader range of health issues that affect women, in line with the local disease burden and trends and in ways that will redress the fragmentation of care that has built up around priority programmes. Improving women's health requires attention to sexual and reproductive health conditions that primarily affect women, but it is also important to deal with other common conditions that remain undetected and untreated in women. For example, women with acute coronary syndromes are often undiagnosed, in part because they often show different symptoms from men. In particular, the growing threat of noncommunicable diseases and mental health problems in women is neglected in many settings. Vision loss causes 32% of years lost due to disability among older women yet they face difficulty in obtaining care.

Third, continuity of care is essential when seeking to address the range of interrelated health problems, both acute and chronic, that affect women over their life course. One of the most serious avoidable risk factors for premature death and disease in adult women is tobacco use. The increasing prevalence of smoking among young women requires urgent action. Starting with the early childhood period and continuing over the years through the promotion of active and healthy ageing, a long-term and comprehensive perspective is needed when investing in the health of women.

Sexual and reproductive health services have often been at the forefront of attempts to promote women-centred care, but these services have tended to focus too narrowly and have missed opportunities to deliver a broader set of interventions or have neglected certain groups of women. For instance, antenatal care should be seen as a potential entry point for a broader package of health services that take into account women's overall health needs.[14] Women living with HIV should have access to disease assessment and treatment for their own sake, and not just for interventions to reduce the risk of transmitting the virus to their infants.[15] Sexual and reproductive health services should also avoid focusing solely on married women and ignoring the needs of unmarried adolescents and marginalized women such as sex workers.

Giving women a voice

There are growing expectations regarding the effective participation of women in the design and implementation of health services that aim to have an impact on their health.[16]

The demand for health services that meet women's needs often comes from organizations working with women or with women's groups at the community level. It is important to work with such organizations and support community participation in planning change. In Nepal a community-based participatory intervention involving women's groups in identifying local birthing problems and formulating strategies to address them has been shown to be effective in reducing maternal and neonatal mortality in a rural population.[17] Community participation has also been successful in organizing transport to health facilities for delivery.[18] These developments in maternal health care for women can lead to far-reaching changes. There is evidence from Malaysia and Sri Lanka that community contacts with skilled midwives as front-line health workers can serve as a basis for expanding a comprehensive health system in rural areas.[19]

It is also essential to empower women who work within the health system at all levels. As noted in Chapter 1, women make up the majority of health workers in most settings but are often excluded from positions of responsibility, thus reflecting more general inequalities in society.[20] A genuine commitment backed up by action is required to increase women's participation at all levels of health governance and particularly in decision-making positions.[21] In the same spirit, women-specific concerns must be mainstreamed through measures such as improved recognition of women-dominated professions (such as nursing), norms and codes of conduct for health workers, supervision (with quality improvements), and pre-service and in-service training and mentoring programmes. Where health workers feel valued, cared for and respected, they are more likely to provide client-centred and better quality services.[22] Finally, it is crucial that steps be taken to prevent the health hazards that female health workers face, including violence in the workplace, and to cater for their health and safety needs.

Approaches to strengthen human resources for health must acknowledge the critical role played by women as informal caregivers in the home and community. It is estimated that up to 80% of all health care and 90% of HIV/AIDS-related illness care is provided in the home.[23] In the context of the HIV/AIDS epidemic, it is generally recognized that women and girls are the principal caregivers and bear the greatest degree of responsibility for the psychosocial and physical care of family and community members.[24] It is vital that these women are given the recognition they deserve and the support they need from the formal and professional sectors – including training, supervision, and functioning referral systems with access to drugs, equipment and skilled expertise.[25]

Universal coverage

A key primary health care reform is equitable access to health care through the provision of universal coverage – i.e. access to a full range of health services, with social health protection for all.

Improving access

Scaling up services towards the provision of universal access represents a major challenge. Progress is patchy and uneven for most of the interventions that could make a difference to the common health problems that affect women. Some services, such as antenatal care, are more likely to be in place than others such as those related to mental health, sexual violence and cervical cancer screening and care.

Most progress is being made by countries that were already in a relatively good position in the early 1990s, whereas those less favourably placed, particularly in sub-Saharan Africa, have been left behind. Stagnation, reversals and slow progress are found mainly in the poorest (and often institutionally the weakest) countries, particularly those affected by conflict or disasters. Aggravating factors specific to conflict and other forms of instability include the disruption of primary health care services and the shortage of health-care providers.[26]

In such contexts, there are very low levels of coverage with basic interventions such as immunization and skilled birth attendance. For many girls and women, the services simply do not exist, or cannot be reached. For example, large numbers of mothers in rural areas are excluded from life-saving care at childbirth simply because of lack of access to hospitals where emergency obstetric care can be provided. Only a small minority of the population enjoys access to a reasonable range of services – leading to a pattern of mass deprivation. At the other extreme are countries where a large part of the population has access to a wide range of services but a minority is excluded - a pattern of marginalization.[27] The barriers to access are many; use of health services is often constrained because of women's lack of decision-making power or the low value placed on women's health.

Documenting and mapping exclusion from various essential services can be a useful tool for planning and can also serve as a baseline against which to measure progress in coverage. In many countries – especially those experiencing stagnation or reversal – the main challenge is to extend the network of health services and build up the range of interventions. In other countries, the determinants of specific patterns of exclusion must be tackled.

Social health protection

Ensuring universal coverage is not just a matter of increasing the supply of services. Financial barriers to the use of services must be eliminated. Universal coverage carries particular significance for women. They face higher health costs than men due to their greater use of health care, and they are also more likely than their male counterparts to be poor, unemployed or else engaged in part-time work or work in the informal sector, which offers no health benefits. Approaches to extending coverage of health care must deal with the content of benefit packages, ensuring that they include a greater range of services for girls and women of all ages. Some countries, such as Thailand, have introduced universal coverage for a comprehensive package of health services, including sexual and reproductive health interventions.[28] Financial protection against the costs of seeking health care must also be addressed – by moving away from user charges and by making prepayment and pooling schemes more common. There is evidence that, where user fees are charged for maternal health services, households pay a substantial proportion of the cost of facility-based services, and the expense of complicated deliveries is often catastrophic. The removal of user fees for maternal health, especially for deliveries, can stimulate demand – as has been seen in Ghana where the government has introduced a policy of free delivery care for all women. Although funding and cash flow problems have been a challenge, evidence indicates an increase in institutional deliveries.[29] Cash transfers (including conditional cash transfers) to women have also been considered as part of a larger package aimed at protecting poor households from cutting back on essential health expenditure during periods of economic downturn.[30–32]

Public policy

Public health policy and practice need to take into account the social context that shapes health for both women and men, and must work towards removing gender-based differentials in accessing health services and achieving positive health outcomes. The health sector also has an important role to play in drawing attention to the ways in which policy in other sectors can affect the health of women, and in encouraging intersectoral collaboration to enhance positive health outcomes for women while minimizing adverse effects.

In view of human rights concerns and international commitments, deliberate action is required to address inequalities.[a] Only if public policy is transformed in ways that empower women, will they be able to reach their full health potential. "Health in all policies" is a call of

a For international commitments that relate to the rights of women, see the Programme of Action adopted at the International Conference on Population and Development, Cairo, 5–13 September 1994 http://www.un.org/popin/icpd/conference/offeng/poa.html; the Beijing Declaration and Platform for Action of the Fourth World Conference on Women, 15 September 1995 http://www.unesco.org/education/information/nfsunesco/pdf/BEIJIN_E.PDF; the International Covenant on Economic, Social and Cultural Rights which was adopted by the United Nations General Assembly on 16 December 1966 and entered into force on 3 January 1976 (http://www2.ohchr.org/english/law/pdf/cescr.pdf); the Convention on the Elimination of All Forms of Discrimination against Women which was adopted by the United Nations General Assembly on 18 December 1979 and entered into force on 3 September 1981 (http://www.un.org/womenwatch/daw/cedaw); and the Convention on the Rights of the Child which was adopted by the United Nations General Assembly on 20 November 1989 and entered into force on 2 September 1990 (http://www2.ohchr.org/english/law/crc.htm).

the renewed movement for primary health care which recognizes that population health can be improved through policies that are mainly controlled by sectors other than health.[33,34]

Women's health in all policies

A range of public policies that impact on the determinants of exposure to risks, disease vulnerability, access to care, and the consequences of ill-health among women is discussed in the background paper of the Women and Gender Equity Knowledge Network of the WHO Commission on Social Determinants of Health. Examples of policy actions that can support progress include:

- legal and social measures that protect women's property rights;[16,35]
- policies that support equal access to formal employment for women as well as gender equality in the workplace, and that protect women against losing promotion, income or job as a result of pregnancy or caring for children and family members;[a]
- targeted action to encourage girls to enrol in and stay in school, by providing school meals, constructing separate sanitation facilities, ensuring a safe school environment and promoting later marriage;[36]
- health promotion and other measures to increase access of all adolescent girls to education, including comprehensive sexuality education, and education and policies on tobacco and alcohol, diet, physical activity, and road safety;
- measures that specifically provide economic opportunities for women, especially in countries that are most vulnerable to the effects of the global economic and food crises;[37]
- measures that increase access to water, fuel and time-saving technologies;
- strategies to challenge gender stereotypes and change discriminatory norms, practices and behaviours;[38]
- action to end all forms of violence against women, including in conflict situations;[39]
- building "age-friendly" environments and increasing opportunities for older women to contribute productively to society, while supporting them in their caring and other roles where needed.

Lessons can be learned from bold national initiatives that have sought to address social inequality and exclusion in ways that promote gender equality and women's health. For example, Chile's multisectoral and integrated approach to social protection for the poor includes a universal programme for early child development. Chile Crece Contigo ("Chile grows with you") includes access to child care, education and health services to help young children achieve their optimal physical, social and emotional development, while enforcing the right of working mothers to nurse their babies and also stimulating women's employment.[40]

Important benefits for women's health can come from social policies that appear to be gender-neutral, such as investments in communications, rural infrastructure and roads, or the upgrading of slums. Lessons may be learned from the persistence of threats to women's health even in high-income countries with strong public health programmes. These include high incidence of sexually transmitted infections, substance use and mental health problems, including suicide. The fact is that a gender analysis is a crucial component of all public policies that are critical to the safeguarding and enhancement of women's health.

---

a For examples of International Labour Conventions that are relevant to this issue, see: Discrimination (Employment and Occupation) Convention (1958), Equal Remuneration Convention (1951), Workers with Family Responsibilities Convention (1981), and Maternity Protection Convention (2000). These conventions are published by the International Labour Organization and can be accessed at http://www.ilo.org/public/english/gender.htm.

Economic opportunities for women

The global financial crisis and economic downturn compounds the difficulties of many countries that are struggling to reach universal coverage of health care. Countries with rapidly decelerating growth, especially those already burdened by high levels of poverty, will find it even harder to fund the provision of health care for those in need. Paradoxically, this situation provides an opportunity to underline the urgency of women's health concerns, and to advocate for the implementation of social and economic measures that will protect the most vulnerable from further economic shocks.

The crisis has already focused attention on the economic empowerment of women as an important component of any policy response. The World Bank has proposed that industrialized countries contribute a percentage of their economic stimulus packages to finance infrastructure projects, social safety net programmes, and micro-financing institutions and small businesses.[41] It has also urged that such efforts should seek to put money in women's hands in poor households because of the large development benefits that will result in terms of mitigating current and future hardship.

Micro-finance schemes have already played an important role in alleviating poverty in certain low-income countries (mainly in South Asia) where women comprise 85% of the poorest 93 million clients of micro-finance institutions.[37] Questions have been raised about the ability of micro-finance to reach the poorest of the poor but there are indications that it is helping women to overcome financial barriers to health care.[42] And there is interest in further exploring its potential to reduce health inequities and to provide a safety net to poor women in settings where universal coverage is not yet in place.

Different approaches have been tried. Micro-credit allows clients to take out loans at low interest rates that can be used to generate income or to pay for services. Micro-credit services for women are increasingly linked with opportunities for training in areas, such as business development, literacy, health and community-building skills, which can lead to a broader range of benefits. A study in South Africa showed, for instance, that a programme that combined micro-credit with gender-based health education halved the risk of intimate partner violence among the participating women.[43] In Bangladesh, health and nutrition benefits have been shown among the women participating in the micro-credit programme of BRAC (Bangladesh Rural Advancement Committee), as well as among their young children.[44]

Micro-insurance and micro-saving schemes are intended to provide some level of health insurance cover, or to encourage women to save for future health needs, or to repay health costs over time. A small health financing experiment in the Indian state of Karnataka included opening a savings account to cover outpatient health-care costs for each woman who was enrolled, plus insurance for inpatient care. More than half of the women's health-care needs were met and the programme's reach was extended to women who had not previously used the formal health system.[45]

Given their potential for women's economic empowerment, and their possible stimulation of health-seeking behaviours, further work is needed to better document and understand the various innovative financing mechanisms that operate at community level. The context in which such schemes flourish, their possible pitfalls, and their potential for replication and sustainability merit more attention. So too, do the ways in which the schemes affect health – particularly the health of poor women in times of economic recession.

Tracking progress

Improvements in planning and implementing policies for women's health and in monitoring results depend on investments in strategic information systems for the collection and use of data disaggregated by sex and age, and the tracking of progress towards global targets and other indicators relevant to women's health and survival.

Currently, reliable data on critical aspects of women's health are not available because of the weakness of country health information and statistical systems. For example, maternal mortality, a powerful indicator both of women's health and the status of a health system, is poorly measured in most low-income settings. To address this deficit and to generate more reliable and timely data on the broader patterns of mortality among both women and men, increased support is needed to build registration systems that identify and count births, deaths and causes of death. While not focused on women's needs per se, this will establish a basis for more accurate monitoring of women's health across the life course.[46]

Women are "more than mothers". Policy-makers have a responsibility to deal with a range of other serious health problems that affect women.[47] A concerted effort is required to better document these issues, many of which are currently invisible or neglected, as highlighted in this report. Better data are also needed for monitoring the performance of the health system in increasing coverage with essential interventions, particularly where inequities are an issue. This work is critical for identifying the various ways in which women and their health are being left behind, whether it be as a result of insufficient progress in improving health, or widening inequalities, or – for some health conditions and in some situations – the emergence of new problems or the worsening of old ones.

Given the major gaps in our knowledge and understanding highlighted in earlier chapters, substantial investments are required in research on women's health issues. The greatest priority should be given to research that will guide, monitor and evaluate action. Women should not be just the subject of study but should be engaged in the research as active participants. Women continue to be excluded from many observational studies and clinical trials, and that must stop. The participation of women and representatives of women's organizations in all steps of the research process is essential for building a more relevant research agenda, bringing fresh insight into the interpretation of research findings, and facilitating relevant changes in policy.

References

1. *Report of the Fourth World Conference on Women, Beijing 4–15 September 1995.* New York, NY, United Nations, 1995. Paragraph 89 (http://www.un.org/womenwatch/daw/beijing/official.htm, accessed 8 April 2009).
2. *The world health report 2008 – primary health care now more than ever.* Geneva, World Health Organization, 2008.
3. Ravindran TKS, Kelkar-Khambete A. Gender mainstreaming in health: looking back, looking forward. *Global Public Health*, 2008, 3 suppl 1;121–142.doi:10.1080/17441690801900761 PMID:19288347
4. Ravindran TKS, Kelkar-Khambete A. *Women's health policies and programmes and gender mainstreaming in health policies, programmes and within the health sector institutions.* Background paper prepared for the Women and Gender Equity Knowledge Network of the WHO Commission on Social Determinants of Health, 2007 (http://www.who.int/social_determinants/resources/womens_health_policies_wgkn_2007.pdf, accessed 10 April 2009).
5. Murthy RK. *Accountability to citizens on gender and health.* Background paper prepared for the Women and Gender Equity Knowledge Network of the WHO Commission on Social Determinants of Health, 2007 (http://www.who.int/social_determinants/resources/accountability_to_citizens_wgkn_2007.pdf, accessed 10 April 2009).
6. *Closing the gap in a generation: health equity through action on the social determinants of health.* Final Report of the Commission on Social Determinants of Health. Geneva, World Health Organization, 2008.
7. Govender V, Penn-Kekana L. *Gender biases and discrimination: a review of health care interpersonal interactions.* Background paper prepared for the Women and Gender Equity Knowledge Network of the WHO Commission on Social Determinants of Health, 2007 (http://www.who.int/social_determinants/resources/gender_biases_and_discrimination_wgkn_2007.pdf, accessed 21 April 2009).
8. Östlin P, Diderichsen F. *Equity-oriented national strategy for public health in Sweden. A case study.* Policy Learning Curve Series No 1. Brussels, European Centre for Health Policy, 2001.
9. Countdown Working Group on Health Policy and Health Systems. Assessment of the health system and policy environment as a critical complement to tracking intervention coverage for maternal, newborn, and child health. *Lancet*, 2008, 371:1284–1293.doi:10.1016/S0140-6736(08)60563-2 PMID:18406863
10. South Africa Every Death Counts Writing Group. Every death counts: use of mortality audit data for decision making to save the lives of mothers, babies, and children in South Africa. *Lancet*, 2008, 371:1294–1304.doi:10.1016/S0140-6736(08)60564-4 PMID:18406864
11. Murthy RK. Strengthening accountability to citizens on gender and health. *Global Public Health*, 2008, 3 suppl 1;104–120.doi:10.1080/17441690801900852 PMID:19288346
12. Matamala M. *The Observatory on Gender Equity in Health in Chile.* Presentation given at the Council of Women World Leaders, Madrid, 2007 (http://www.realizingrights.org/pdf/MLI_Madrid_Meeting_Report_April_2007.pdf, accessed 20 April 2009).
13. Gijsbers Van Wijk CMT, Van Vliet KP, Kolk AM. Gender perspectives and quality of care: towards appropriate and adequate health care. *Social Science & Medicine*, 1996, 43:707–720. doi:10.1016/0277-9536(96)00115-3 PMID:8870135
14. Rosenfield A, Maine D. Maternal mortality- a neglected tragedy: where is the M in MCH? *Lancet*, 1985, 326:83–85.doi:10.1016/S0140-6736(85)90188-6
15. Rosenfield A, Figdor E. Where is the M in MTCT? The broader issues in mother-to-child transmission of HIV. *American Journal of Public Health*, 2001, 91:703–704.doi:10.2105/AJPH.91.5.703 PMID:11344873
16. Sen G, Östlin P. *Unequal, unfair, ineffective and inefficient. Gender inequity in health: why it exists and how we can change it.* Final report to the Women and Gender Equity Knowledge Network of the WHO Commission on Social Determinants of Health. 2007 (http://www.who.int/social_determinants/resources/csdh_media/wgekn_final_report_07.pdf, accessed 14 April 2009).

17. Manandhar DS et al. Effect of a participatory intervention with women's groups on birth outcomes in Nepal: cluster-randomised controlled trial. *Lancet*, 2004, 364:970–979.doi:10.1016/S0140-6736(04)17021-9 PMID:15364188

18. Ahluwalia IB, Schmid T, Kouletio M, Kanenda O. An evaluation of a community-based approach to safe motherhood in northwestern Tanzania. *International Journal of Gynaecology and Obstetrics: the Official Organ of the International Federation of Gynaecology and Obstetrics*, 2003, 82:231–240.doi:10.1016/S0020-7292(03)00081-X PMID:12873791

19. Pathmanathan I et al. *Investing in maternal health. Learnings from Malaysia and Sri Lanka*. Washington, DC, The World Bank, 2003.

20. George A. Nurses, community health workers, and home carers: gendered human resources compensating for skewed health systems Global. *Public Health*, 2008, 3 S1;75–89. PMID:19288344

21. Brown H, Reichenbach L. *Increasing health systems performance: gender and the global health workforce*. Presentation at the Global Forum for Health Research, Forum 8, Mexico, November 2004.

22. Govender V, Penn-Kekana L. Gender biases and discrimination: a review of health care interpersonal interactions. *Global Public Health*, 2008, 3 suppl 1;90–103. doi:10.1080/17441690801892208 PMID:19288345

23. Uys L. Guest editorial. Longer-term aid to combat AIDS. *Journal of Advanced Nursing*, 2003, 44:1–2.doi:10.1046/j.1365-2648.2003.02787.x PMID:12956663

24. Ogden J, Esim S, Grown C. Expanding the care continuum for HIV/Aids: bringing carers into focus. *Health Policy and Planning*, 2006, 21:333–342.doi:10.1093/heapol/czl025 PMID:16940299

25. Sen G, Iyer A, George A. Systematic hierarchies and systemic failures: gender and health inequities in Koppal District. *Economic and Political Weekly*, 2007, 42:682–690.

26. *Health action in crises: annual report 2008 – primary health care in crises*. Geneva, World Health Organization, 2009.

27. *The world health report 2005: make every mother and child count*. Geneva, World Health Organization, 2005.

28. Tangcharoensathien V et al. Universal coverage and its impact on reproductive health services in Thailand. *Reproductive Health Matters*, 2002, 10:59–69.doi:10.1016/S0968-8080(02)00087-3 PMID:12557643

29. Borghi J et al. Mobilising financial resources for maternal health. *Lancet*, 2006, 368:1457–1465. doi:10.1016/S0140-6736(06)69383-5 PMID:17055948

30. Doetinchem O, Xu K, Carrin G. *Conditional cash transfers: what's in it for health?* Technical Brief for Policy-Makers No 1/2008. Geneva, World Health Organization, 2008 (http://www.who.int/entity/health_financing/documents/pb_e_08_1-cct.pdf, accessed 16 April 2009).

31. Brandstetter RH. *Evaluation of OFDA cash for relief intervention in Ethiopia*. Washington, DC, United States Agency for International Development /Office of US Foreign Disaster Assistance, 2004 (http://pdf.dec.org/pdf_docs/Pdacd354.pdf, accessed 16 April 2009).

32. *Potential applications of conditional cash transfers for prevention of sexually transmitted infections and HIV in sub-Saharan Africa*. Policy research working paper No. 4673. Washington, DC, The World Bank, 2008 (http://www-wds.worldbank.org/external/default/WDSContentServer/IW3P/IB/2008/07/22/000158349_20080722084441/Rendered/PDF/WPS4673.pdf, accessed 17 April 2009).

33. Stahl T et al., eds. *Health in all policies: prospects and potentials*. Oslo, Ministry of Social Affairs and Health, 2006.

34. Puska P. Health in all policies. *European Journal of Public Health*, 2007, 17:328.doi:10.1093/eurpub/ckm048 PMID:17553811

35. *To have and to hold: women's property and inheritance rights in the context of HIV/AIDS in sub-Saharan Africa*. Washington, DC, International Center for Research on Women, 2004 (http://www.icrw.org/docs/2004_paper_haveandhold.pdf, accessed 17 April 2009).

36. United Nations Girls' Education Initiative. New York, NY, United Nations Children's Fund (UNICEF) (http://www.ungei.org/whatisungei/index.html, accessed 16 April 2009).

37. *The global financial crisis; assessing vulnerability for women and children.* Policy Brief. Washington, DC, The World Bank, 2009 (http://www.worldbank.org/html/extdr/financialcrisis/pdf/Women-Children-Vulnerability-March09.pdf, accessed 30 March 2009).

38. Keleher H, Franklin L. Changing gendered norms about women and girls at the level of household and community: a review of the evidence. *Global Public Health*, 2008, 3 suppl 1;42–57. PMID:19288342

39. *In-depth study on all forms of violence against women. Report of the Secretary-General.* Document submitted to the Sixty-first session of the United Nations General Assembly, July 2006. Document No. A/61/122/Add.1 6. New York, NY, United Nations, 2006 (http://www.un.org/womenwatch/daw/vaw/v-sg-study.htm, accessed 21 April 2009).

40. Frenz P. *Innovative practices for intersectoral action on health: a case study of four programs for social equity. Chilean case study prepared for the CSDH.* Santiago, Ministry of Health, Division of Health and Family Planning, Social Determinants of Health Initiative, 2007.

41. *Zoellick calls for 'Vulnerability Fund' ahead of Davos Forum.* News announcement 30 January 2009. Washington, DC, The World Bank, 2009 (http://web.worldbank.org/WBSITE/EXTERNAL/NEWS/0,contentMDK:22049582~pagePK:64257043~piPK:437376~theSitePK:4607,00.html, accessed 23 June 2009).

42. Mohindra K, Haddad S, Narayana D. Can microcredit help improve the health of poor women? Some findings from a cross-sectional study in Kerala, India. *International Journal for Equity in Health*, 2008, 7:2.doi:10.1186/1475-9276-7-2 PMID:18186918

43. Pronyk PM et al. Effect of a structural intervention for the prevention of intimate-partner violence and HIV in rural South Africa: a cluster randomised trial. *Lancet*, 2006, 368:1973–1983. doi:10.1016/S0140-6736(06)69744-4 PMID:17141704

44. Chowdhury AM, Bhuiya A. Do poverty alleviation programmes reduce inequities in health? The Bangladesh experience. In: Leon D, Walt G, eds. *Poverty, inequality and health.* Oxford, Oxford University Press, 2001:312–332.

45. Durairaj V et al. *Shaping national health financing systems: can micro-banking contribute?* Technical Brief for Policy Makers No 2/2009. Geneva, World Health Organization, 2009 (http://www.who.int/health_financing/documents/cov-pb_e_09_2-microbanking/en/index.html, accessed 9 April 2009).

46. AbouZahr C et al. The way forward. "Who counts?" series, No. 4. *Lancet*, 2007, 370:1791–1799. doi:10.1016/S0140-6736(07)61310-5 PMID:18029003

47. Women: more than mothers [Editorial]. *Lancet*, 2007, 370:1283.doi:10.1016/S0140-6736(07)61546-3 PMID:17933626

CONCLUSION

Conclusion

This global overview shows that while the health of girls and women has much improved over the past 60 years, the gains have been unevenly spread. In many parts of the world, women's lives, from childhood to old age, are diminished by preventable illness and premature death. This year, more than four million girls under the age of five will die from conditions that can, for the most part, be prevented or treated. More than 2.5 million elderly women will go blind for reasons that are similarly avoidable. Between these extremes of the human lifespan, a million women will die from HIV/AIDS, half a million from tuberculosis, and another half a million from complications related to pregnancy and childbirth.

This report highlights the commonalities in the health challenges facing women around the world but also draws attention to the differences that arise from the varied circumstances in which they live. The report makes the case that addressing women's health is a necessary and effective approach to strengthening health systems overall – action that will benefit everyone. Primary health care – with its focus on equity, solidarity and social justice – offers an opportunity to make a difference.

A startling fact that emerges from the report is the paucity of reliable data. Even maternal mortality, one of the most egregious threats to women's health in the developing world, remains poorly measured. There are gaps in our understanding of the way that most health threats affect females as distinct from males, and of the differential effects on girls and women of health interventions and services. Not enough is known about how health systems should be structured and managed to respond effectively to the particular needs of girls and women – especially the poorest and most vulnerable among them. Thus this report is also a call for better data, for more research, for more systematic monitoring of the health of the female half of the world, and for addressing the barriers that girls and women face in protecting their health and in accessing health care and information.

In reviewing the evidence and setting an agenda for the future, this report points the way towards the actions needed to improve the health of girls and women. The report aims to inform policy dialogue and stimulate action by countries, agencies and development partners.

Improving women's health matters to women, to their families, and to communities and societies at large.

Improve women's health – improve the world.

Index

Page numbers in italic indicate figures and tables